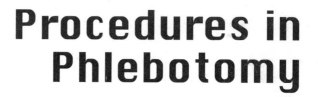

Procedures in Phlebotomy

Second Edition

John C. Flynn, Jr., PhD, MS, MT(ASCP), SBB
Professor and Chairman, Division of Allied Health
and Physical Education
Director, Medical Laboratory Technician and
Phlebotomy Programs
Montgomery County Community College
Blue Bell, Pennsylvania

W.B. SAUNDERS COMPANY

An Imprint of Elsevier Science

Philadelphia London New York St. Louis Sydney Toronto

W.B. SAUNDERS COMPANY
An Imprint of Elsevier Science

The Curtis Center
Independence Square West
Philadelphia, Pennsylvania 19106

Library of Congress Cataloging-in-Publication Data

Flynn, John C.
    Procedures in phlebotomy / John C. Flynn, Jr. — 2nd ed.
        p.   cm.
    Rev. ed. of: Procedures in phlebotomy / edited by John C. Flynn, Jr.
c1994.
    Includes bibliographical references and index.
    ISBN 0–7216–7583–2
    1. Phlebotomy. I. Title.
    [DNLM: 1. Phlebotomy–methods. 2. Blood Specimen Collection—
methods. WB 381 F648p 1999]
    RM182.P76 1999
    616.07′561—dc21
    DNLM/DLC   98–43926

PROCEDURES IN PHLEBOTOMY, 2nd edition   ISBN 0–7216–7583–2

Printed in the United States of America

Last digit is the print number: 9   8   7   6   5

I would like to dedicate this book to my wife, Mary Ellen, and our children, Meghan, Mary Ellen, Jack, Eamonn, Rory, and Brighid.

Contributors

Georganne K. Buescher, Med, MS, EdD

Associate Dean, College of Graduate Studies and Clinical Assistant
Professor, Department of Microbiology and Immunology
Thomas Jefferson University
Director of Master of Science Programs
College of Graduate Studies
Thomas Jefferson University
Philadelphia, Pennsylvania
Infectious Diseases and Their Prevention

Beth V. Dronson, BS, VMD

Professor, Veterinary Technology Program
Manor Junior College
Jenkintown, Pennsylvania
Staff Veterinarian
Warminster Veterinary Hospital
Warminster, Pennsylvania
Green Lane Veterinary Hospital
Green Lane, Pennsylvania
Animal Phlebotomy

Debra Lynn Eckman, MS, MT(ASCP)

Instructor, MLT Program
Montgomery County Community College
Blue Bell, Pennsylvania
Medical Technologist
Phoenixville Hospital
Phoenixville, Pennsylvania
Anatomy and Physiology

Shirley E. Greening, MS, JD, CFIAC

Chairman and Professor
Department of Laboratory Sciences
Program Director, Cytotechnology
Coordinator of Health Policy
Center for Collaborative Research
College of Health Professions
Thomas Jefferson University
Philadelphia, Pennsylvania
 Medical-Legal Issues and Health Law Procedures

Joyce E. Hill, BA, MT(ASCP)

Instructor, MLT Program
Montgomery County Community College
Blue Bell, Pennsylvania
Medical Technologist
Grand View Hospital
Sellersville, Pennsylvania
Instructor—Medical Assistants
Lansdale School of Business
North Wales, Pennsylvania
 Multiskilling for Phlebotomists

Maryann D. Harrison, MHA, MT(ASCP)

Technical Manager, Outpatient Laboratory/Phlebotomy
Hospital of the University of Pennsylvania
Philadelphia, Pennsylvania
 Total Quality in Phlebotomy Service

Mary P. Nix, MS, MT(ASCP), SBB

Technical Supervisor, Blood Bank
Hospital of the University of Pennsylvania
Philadelphia, Pennsylvania
 Total Quality in Phlebotomy Service

Dorothy Pfender, BA, MT, BSS

Instructor, MLT Program
Montgomery County Community College
Blue Bell, Pennsylvania
 Phlebotomy Department Management

Preface

A s with the first edition, this second edition of *Procedures in Phlebotomy* is intended for students of phlebotomy. These students may be just entering the field or they may have been practicing the art of blood collection for many years. Whomever wishes to remain abreast of this rapidly changing and expanding field will find this book useful.

This edition is still divided into two sections but there are many enhancements. The Anatomy and Physiology chapter is expanded with more relevant information for phlebotomists. The Infectious Disease chapter has numerous updates including expanded hepatitis discussion, TB discussion, and standard precautions. Chapters 4, 5, and 6, the crucial phlebotomy chapters, include updated equipment and numerous new and redone photographs. Chapter 8 is completely new and discusses the role of multiskilling for phlebotomists. The Animal Phlebotomy chapter can now be found as an appendix. The Phlebotomy Department Management chapter has been thoroughly updated, as has the Total Quality in Phlebotomy Service chapter.

Additionally, the glossary has expanded by 20 percent. Terms in the glossary are still noted as boldfaced terms in the text. The review examination now has 120 questions and most chapters have additional review questions. A color review chart is still included with additional information. With all these enhancements and additions, I am sure students and instructors will find this text more useful than ever.

Acknowledgments

M any people, both formally and informally, contributed to this second edition. The contributors were, without a doubt, crucial to this book. Marge Johnson contributed in ways too numerous to list in this space. Barbara Proud, the photographer, was outstanding and a pleasure to work with. The team at W.B. Saunders Company was especially helpful and very supportive. Lastly, I would like to thank Selma Kaszczuk, whom I will miss.

Contents

CHAPTER

4 Equipment 69

John C. Flynn, Jr.

CHAPTER

5 Proper Procedures for Venipuncture 87
John C. Flynn, Jr.

CHAPTER

6 Special Collection Procedures 115
John C. Flynn, Jr.

CHAPTER

7 Complications of Phlebotomy 135
John C. Flynn, Jr.

CHAPTER

PART 2

Professional Issues / 165

CHAPTER

CHAPTER

10 Phlebotomy Department Management 179
Dorothy Pfender

CHAPTER

11 Total Quality in Phlebotomy Service 195
Mary P. Nix and Maryann D. Harrison

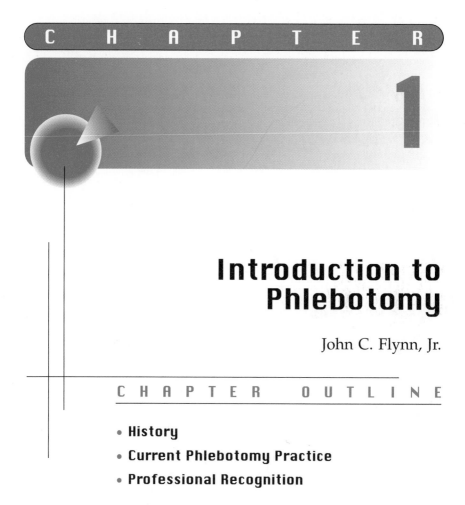

Introduction to Phlebotomy

John C. Flynn, Jr.

C H A P T E R   O U T L I N E

- **History**
- **Current Phlebotomy Practice**
- **Professional Recognition**

HISTORY

"Bleed in the acute affections, if the disease appear strong, and the patients be in the vigor of life, and if they have strength." These were the thoughts of Hippocrates, recorded nearly 25 centuries ago, regarding the usefulness of **phlebotomy.** He proposed that phlebotomy be used as a treatment for acute disease conditions.

Later, during the eleventh century, when the first school of medicine was founded in Salerno in present-day Italy, "blood letting" was still a popular curative. In fact, well into modern times (that is, the seventeenth and eighteenth centuries), phlebotomy was used as a treatment for diseases ranging from mental illness to fever to convulsions (Fig. 1–1). However, as the practice of medicine and the understanding of the

3

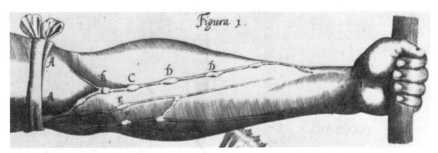

FIGURE 1-1 • Drawing depicting the location of veins in the arm originally published in 1628. (From Harvey, W. [1628]. Exercitio anatomica de mortu cordis et sanguinis in animalibus. Frankfurt: G. Fitzer, 1628. Courtesy of the Wellcome Institute Library, London.)

human body progressed, phlebotomy as a routine treatment fell into disuse.

CURRENT PHLEBOTOMY PRACTICE

Today, phlebotomy, although no longer considered a curative, is a necessary aid in the diagnosis and treatment of disease. In ancient times, witch doctors, barbers, and, later, physicians performed phlebotomies (Fig. 1–2), but in modern times trained professionals perform this vital function. These professionals, who traditionally were trained on the job, are increasingly being trained in formal programs and becoming certified by national certifying agencies (Table 1–1).

With the growth of modern medicine and the increasingly wide range of diagnostic and screening tests available, the role of the phlebotomist has become increasingly important and complex. Table 1–2 lists primary sections and the tests common to most clinical laboratories. The list of tests is not all inclusive, but gives the reader a sampling of the hundreds of assays performed in a laboratory. No longer is it a matter of simply collecting a blood specimen; the modern phlebotomist must also be aware of the type of test requested, any medications the patient is taking that may interfere with the testing, the importance of the timing of the blood collection, and the effect of the patient's diet.

The modern phlebotomist may also be called on to perform other functions such as measuring bleeding times, collecting donor blood, performing therapeutic phlebotomies and bedside testing, and preparing specimens. Phlebotomists today must communicate and interact with the entire laboratory team (Fig. 1–3A). They must be familiar with both routine and special specimen requirements, including collection and transportation procedures for each section of the laboratory. Lately, due to changes in health care management, phlebotomists are being called upon

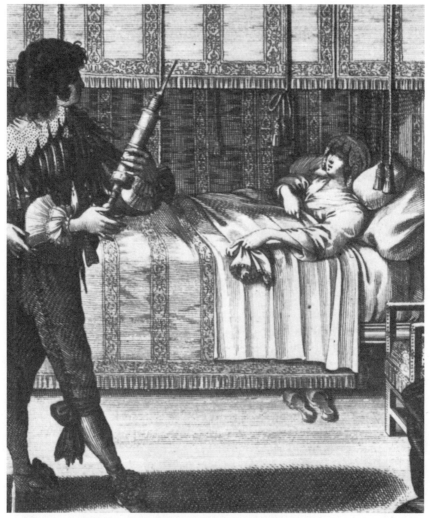

FIGURE 1-2 • Abraham Bosse's *The Physician's Visit*. (Reproduced by Courtesy of the Trustees of the British Museum, London.)

TABLE 1-1 • Phlebotomy Certifying Agencies

American Association of Allied Health Professionals, Inc. (AAAHP)
American Medical Technologists (AMT)
American Society of Clinical Pathologists (ASCP)
American Society of Phlebotomy Technicians (ASPT)
National Credentialing Agency for Laboratory Personnel (NCA)
National Phlebotomy Association (NPA)

TABLE 1–2 • **Common Tests in the Primary Sections
of a Clinical Laboratory**

Hematology
    Complete blood count (CBC)
    White blood cell differential
    Protime (PT)
    Activated partial thromboplastin time (APTT)

Chemistry
    Chemistry profiles
    Glucose
    Cholesterol
    Electrolytes
    Bilirubin
    Blood urea nitrogen (BUN)
    Creatinine
    Enzymes
    Urinalysis (may be in hematology)

Microbiology and Serology
    Gram stains
    Plating of culture
    Sensitivity testing
    Pregnancy tests
    Monospots
    Rheumatoid arthritis screen
    Rapid plasmin reagent (RPR)
    C-reactive protein

Blood Bank
    Blood types
    Antibody screening
    Prenatal testing

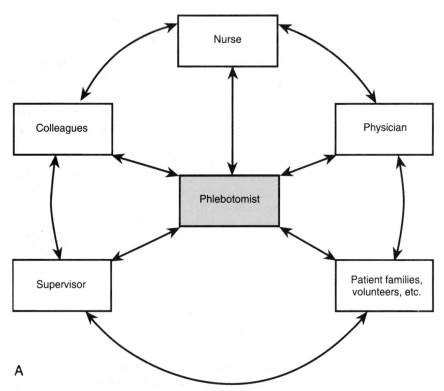

A

FIGURE 1–3 • *A,* A phlebotomist's hospital communication network.

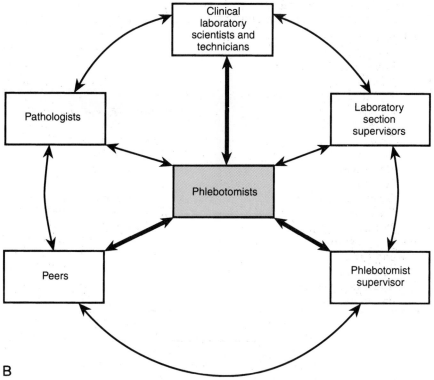

FIGURE 1-3 • *Continued. B,* A phlebotomist's laboratory communication network. The heavier lines indicate more frequent communication pathways.

to perform such tests as **electrocardiographs,** simple laboratory tests and some nursing functions to name a few. This process is known as cross-training or multiskilling. See Chapter 8.

Additionally, phlebotomists must also interact and communicate with the entire health care team as well as with patients' families (Fig. 1–3*B*). This means they must be able to "speak the language" of medicine and communicate professionally, both in writing and orally.

Furthermore, phlebotomists are not confined to working exclusively in a hospital setting. They may work in physician office laboratories, blood collection centers such as those operated by the American Red Cross, research institutes, commercial laboratories, or veterinary offices.

PROFESSIONAL RECOGNITION

Figure 1–4 illustrates the organizational structure of modern laboratories, with the position of the phlebotomist highlighted; it can be seen

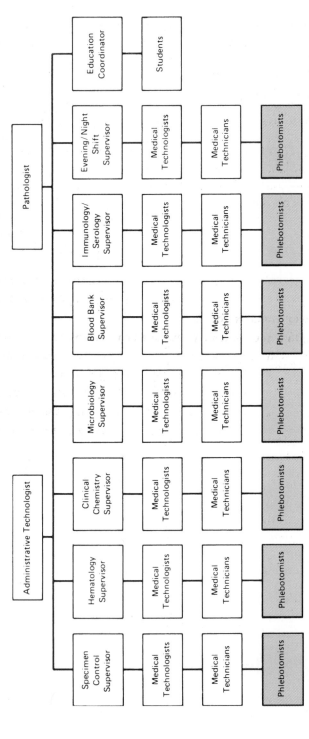

FIGURE 1-4 • Organizational structure of a clinical laboratory. (From Garza D, Becan-McBride K. Phlebotomy Handbook. 3rd ed. Norwalk, CT, Appleton & Lange, p. 13.)

that phlebotomists are an integral part of every laboratory section and play a vital role in the health maintenance team. This partially explains the increasing number of phlebotomy training programs and the increasing number of phlebotomists becoming certified. Currently there are more than 40 approved phlebotomy programs in the United States, with more than 15,000 phlebotomists certified. As has been shown in Table 1–1, there are several different accrediting agencies that certify phlebotomists, and although the examination fees and frequency of examination administration may vary, the underlying goal of all such programs is the same: to assure employers that the phlebotomists they are hiring meet a minimally acceptable standard of practice.

Finally, all professionals should adhere to a code of conduct or a code of ethics. Early physicians followed the Hippocratic oath, and although there is no specific oath or code for phlebotomists, there is one for the field of medical technology, to which phlebotomists belong. This code is endorsed by the American Society for Clinical Laboratory Science:

Being fully cognizant of my responsibilities in the practice of Medical Technology, I affirm my willingness to discharge my duties with accuracy, thoughtfulness and care.

Realizing that the knowledge obtained concerning patients in the course of my work must be treated as confidential, I hold inviolate the confidence placed in me by patients and physicians.

Recognizing that my integrity and that of my profession must be pledged to the absolute reliability on my work, I will conduct myself at all times in a manner appropriate to the dignity of my profession.

REVIEW QUESTIONS

1. Phlebotomy is a necessary aid in the _DIAGNOSIS_ and _TREATMENT_ of disease.
2. Before formal phlebotomy training programs existed, phlebotomists were trained _ON THE JOB_
3. Name some places other than hospitals that may employ phlebotomists.
4. What is the purpose of certification for phlebotomists?
5. A code of conduct that can apply to phlebotomists is published by the _American Society For Medical Technology_

Bibliography

Castiglioni A: A history of medicine. New York, Jason Aronson, 1969.
Haggard HW: Devils, drugs, and doctors. New York, Harper and Brothers, 1929.
Hippocrates: The theory and practice of medicine. New York, Philosophical Library, 1964.
Inglis BA: A history of medicine. Cleveland, The World Publishing Company, 1965.

2

Anatomy and Physiology

Debra Lynn Eckman

The human organism is the most fascinating scientific entity that exists. It can be studied from several perspectives including anatomical, physiological, psychological, and sociological. It can be studied from the simple level of atoms and molecules to the most complex level of the total organism—the living individual. This chapter will explore the anatomy and physiology pertinent to phlebotomists.

BODY PLANES AND CELLS

The parts of the body are studied relative to the planes, or imaginary flat surfaces, that pass through the body (Fig. 2–1). It is important to become familiar with these planes so one can understand the anatomical relationship of one body or organ part to another. The sagittal plane divides the body or an organ into right and left sides. If this plane passes through the midline or center of the body or organ, it is called the midsaggital or median plane. If it divides the organ into unequal right and left sides, it is called the parasagittal plane. A frontal or coronal plane divides the body or organ into front (anterior) and back (posterior) portions. A transverse plane divides the body or organ into top (superior) and bottom (posterior) portions.

Additionally, while the body can be "divided" into sections, there are several levels of organization within the structural framework of the human body (Fig. 2–2). Atoms combine with each other to form molecules. Molecules join with each other to form cells. Cells are the smallest, most basic unit of life. Each type of cell has its own structure and each performs a different function to enable growth, metabolism, transportation, and reproduction within the human body. Cells are generally classified into two groups: somatic cells, which comprise body mass, and gonadal cells, which are vital for reproduction. Similar cells that work together to perform a particular function are called tissues. The study of cells is cytology and the study of tissues is histology.

TISSUES

Tissues within the body are classified into four types based on their function and structure:

1. Epithelial tissue forms the outer layer of skin and some internal organs and the inner lining of blood vessels. Additionally, epithelial cells line body cavities and interior structures within the body's systems. The secreting portion of glands is also composed of epithelial tissue.

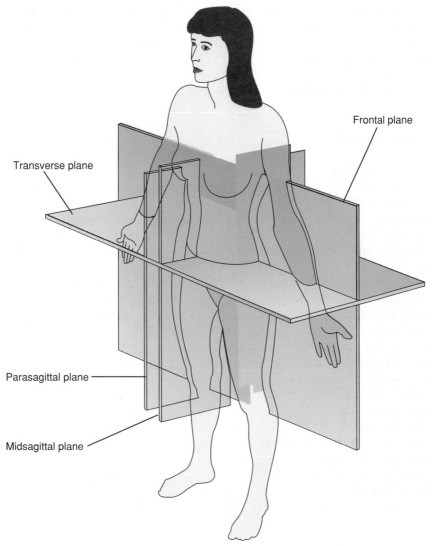

FIGURE 2-1 • Planes of the human body.

2. Connective tissue supports and protects the body and its organs. It aids in binding organs together while also providing immunity and energy storage in the form of fat or adipose tissue. **Cartilage** and bone are examples of connective tissue.

3. Muscle tissue consists of fibers (cells), provides motion, and helps the body maintain posture. It forms the walls of internal organs such as the stomach, heart, and blood vessels.

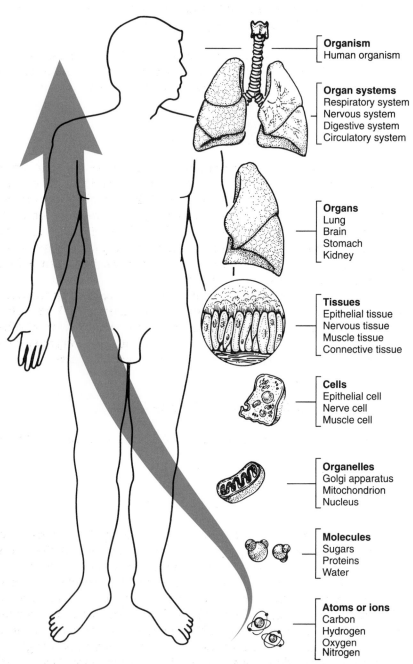

Organism
Human organism

Organ systems
Respiratory system
Nervous system
Digestive system
Circulatory system

Organs
Lung
Brain
Stomach
Kidney

Tissues
Epithelial tissue
Nervous tissue
Muscle tissue
Connective tissue

Cells
Epithelial cell
Nerve cell
Muscle cell

Organelles
Golgi apparatus
Mitochondrion
Nucleus

Molecules
Sugars
Proteins
Water

Atoms or ions
Carbon
Hydrogen
Oxygen
Nitrogen

FIGURE 2-2 • Levels of organization of the human body.

4. Nervous tissue consists of complex, specialized cells (neurons) that transmit nerve impulses to tissues, glands, or other neurons throughout the body to help coordinate body activities.

Each organ in the body is composed of different combinations of these tissues. For example, the stomach—made mostly of epithelial and muscle tissues—contains lesser amounts of other tissues as well.

ORGAN SYSTEMS

The study of anatomy and physiology (structure and function of the body) concentrates on the study of body systems. A body system consists of several related organs that work together to perform a common function. For example, the circulatory system, which is composed of the heart and blood vessels, provides the body with nourishment by circulating blood and nutrients through it. Usually, the organs of a system are anatomically connected; however, in some cases the tissues are widely distributed as seen in the endocrine system.

Body systems work together continuously and constantly interact to maintain a state of internal balance known as homeostasis. A disruption of this homeostasis as caused by one organ or system may affect other organ systems within the body. We will discuss each of the organ systems with emphasis on the cardiovascular and respiratory systems.

DESCRIPTIONS OF THE ORGAN SYSTEMS

In the following discussion, organ systems are grouped according to their main functions.

THE INTEGUMENTARY SYSTEM

The integumentary system, which covers the body, consists of the skin and accessory structures (Fig. 2–3). The skin, one of the largest organs in the body, consists of two principal layers. The thin, outer layer of the skin is the epidermis. Beneath this is the thicker connective tissue, or dermis, which rests on the subcutaneous layer that is composed of additional connective and adipose tissue. Fibers from the dermis connect the skin to the subcutaneous layer. The subcutaneous layer then attaches to tissues and organs. Hair follicles, nails, nerve endings, sweat glands, and **sebaceous glands** are also included in the integumentary system. This system aids in the regulation of body temperature, provides a physical protective barrier against bacteria and dehydration, contains

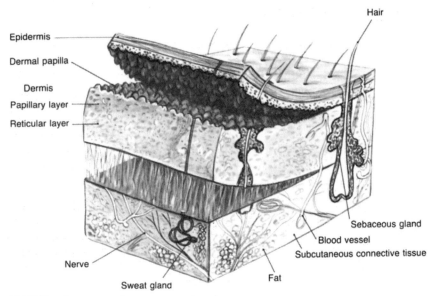

Hair
Epidermis
Dermal papilla
Dermis
Papillary layer
Reticular layer
Sebaceous gland
Blood vessel
Subcutaneous connective tissue
Nerve
Fat
Sweat gland

FIGURE 2-3 • Cross section of the skin. (From Dienhart CM: Basic Human Anatomy and Physiology. 3rd ed. Philadelphia, PA, WB Saunders, 1979, p. 26.)

receptors to touch and pain, houses blood vessels for circulation, and assists in the production of vitamin D within the body. The external location of the integumentary system's structures helps physicians diagnose disease because abnormalities can be easily observed. Dermatology is the medical specialty that pertains to the treatment of skin and related disorders.

SYSTEMS NEEDED FOR MOVEMENT AND SUPPORT

The Skeletal System

The bones of the skeleton (Fig. 2–4) are divided into axial and appendicular portions. The axial portion consists of the skull (cranial and facial bones), vertebral column, and thorax (sternum and ribs). The appendicular portion consists of the shoulder girdle, pelvic (hip) girdle, and bones of the upper (arm) and lower (leg) extremities. There are 80 bones in the axial portion and 126 bones in the appendicular portion of the skeleton. The skeletal system provides the framework of the body, protects vital organs, and works with the muscular system to produce movement. Blood cells are produced within the red marrow of the bones. Orthopedics is the medical specialty that studies the skeletal system and associated structures.

The Muscular System

Muscle tissue is differentiated by its appearance, location, and function. There are three types of muscle tissue:

1. **Smooth muscle** tissue (visceral) is located in the walls of blood vessels and hollow organs such as the stomach. This tissue looks smooth or nonstriated because it lacks alternating light- and dark-colored bands. It is involuntary muscle tissue, which means it needs stimulation from hormones or nerve transmitter substances to function.

2. **Cardiac muscle** tissue forms most of the heart. This tissue is striated because it has varying bands and is involuntary. The contraction of this muscle is usually not under the body's conscious control and is responsible for the heart's ability to beat.

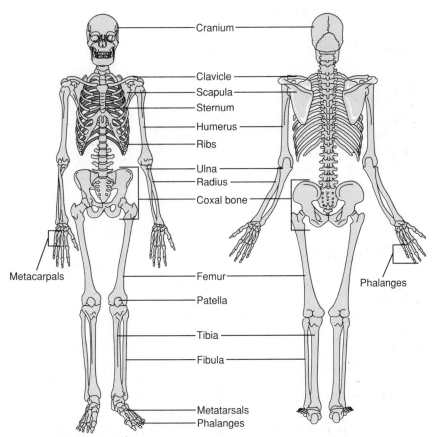

FIGURE 2-4 • Anterior and posterior view of the skeletal system.

3. **Skeletal muscle** tissue primarily attaches itself to the bones and helps to move the skeleton. It is striated and voluntary because it can be made to contract and relax with conscious control.

There are more than 700 muscles in the body (Figs. 2–5*A*, 2–5*B*). Muscles need a source of energy to function. For example, glucose from the blood enters the contracting muscle. Oxygen releases the energy from the glucose and it is converted to the energy form ATP **(Adenosine Triphosphate).** Calcium then interacts with the contractile filaments within the muscle cells. Oxygen is not always required for muscle function; however, if this **anaerobic** process continues for an extended period of time, **lactic acid** accumulates in the blood and muscle tissue. This buildup soon causes muscle fatigue. As skeletal muscle contracts to work, heat is generated. Much of the heat is used to maintain normal

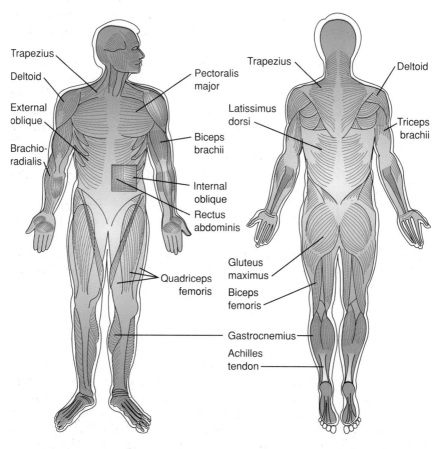

A Anterior view   B Posterior view

FIGURE 2-5 • The muscular system.

body temperature. For example, a football player helps to keep his body warm by actively participating in the sport even in very cold weather. Myology is the study of muscles.

SYSTEMS THAT CONTROL AND COORDINATE ACTIVITIES

The Nervous System

The purpose of the nervous system is to detect changes, known as stimuli, from both internal and external environments. It then analyzes the information and coordinates an appropriate response. Nerve cells, or neurons, conduct impulses from the receptors in the body to and within the central nervous system (CNS). The body also uses chemicals called neurotransmitters to carry impulses between neurons. A common neurotransmitter is acetylcholine. The junction between two neurons is called a synapse.

The nervous system is divided into two sections (Fig. 2–6). The CNS consists of the brain and spinal cord. The peripheral nervous system (PNS) consists of all nervous tissue outside the CNS. The PNS is further divided into the somatic nervous system (SNS) and the autonomic nervous system (ANS) (Fig. 2–7). The SNS conveys information from the head, body wall, and extremities to the CNS. The CNS then sends impulses to the skeletal muscle. The ANS conveys information from the viscera to the CNS. The CNS then sends impulses to the stomach and cardiac muscle and glands.

The ANS is further divided into two systems: the sympathetic and the parasympathetic. The sympathetic system stimulates or excites the organ to start activity. This is known as the "fight or flight" response. The parasympathetic system decreases or inhibits activity to restore and maintain balance. Neurology is the medical specialty that studies the nervous system.

The Sensory System

The sensory system, a component of the nervous system, contains many receptor cells that can detect stimuli. The receptors may be widely distributed or localized in the sense organs within the body. The sense organs include the eye, ear, tongue, and nose. They are responsible for vision, hearing and equilibrium, taste, and smell, respectively. General receptors detect touch, pain, pressure, and temperature. The medical specialties that diagnose abnormalities within this system include ophthalmology (eyes) and otolaryngology (ears, nose, and throat).

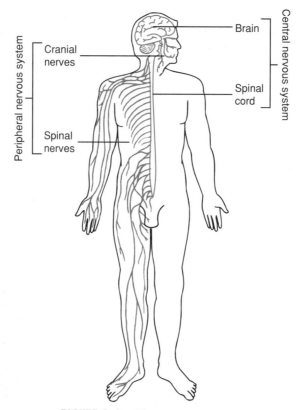

FIGURE 2-6 • The nervous system.

The Endocrine System

The body contains two types of glands that secrete substances that affect other cells: exocrine and endocrine. Exocrine glands secrete substances into ducts that are then carried to organs, body cavities, or outside the body. Sweat glands are an example of this type. The remainder of the discussion will be devoted to endocrine glands which constitute the endocrine system. Endocrine glands secrete their substances or **hormones** into the space around the secretory cells. Examples of these glands include the **pituitary** which is regulated by the **hypothalamus** in the brain, the **thyroid** which is located below the **larynx** or voice box, and the **adrenals** which lie superior to each of the kidneys. Figure 2–8 shows the major endocrine glands.

Hormones are very powerful substances. They regulate metabolism and energy production, contraction of muscles, growth, and aspects of the immune system. They also help to maintain homeostasis within the body and play an important role in the reproductive cycle from its initial stages of gamete production through delivery of the newborn infant. Prolactin, insulin, and oxytocin are just a few of the many hormones secreted in the human body. Endocrinology is the study of the endocrine system.

SYSTEMS THAT TRANSPORT MATERIALS

The Cardiovascular System

All cells within the body must be constantly supplied with nutrients and oxygen. The circulatory system (Fig. 2–9) is responsible for this function. It also removes waste products and carbon dioxide by trans-

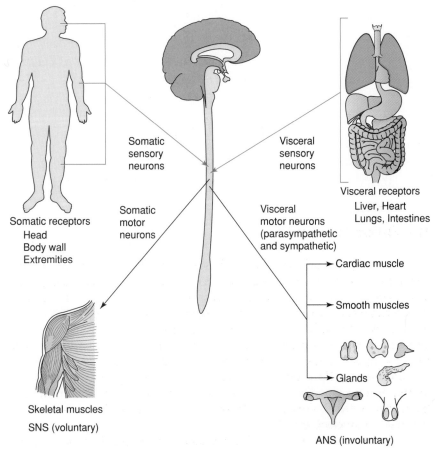

FIGURE 2-7 • The somatic nervous system and autonomic nervous system.

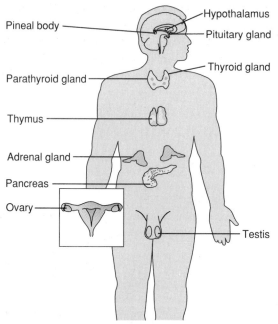

Pineal body
Hypothalamus
Pituitary gland
Thyroid gland
Parathyroid gland
Thymus
Adrenal gland
Pancreas
Ovary
Testis

FIGURE 2-8 • The endocrine system.

porting them to the proper sites for disposal. Additionally, it helps to control body temperature. The circulatory system consists of the heart which pumps blood through blood vessels. The lymphatic vessels return **lymph,** which is very similar to interstitial fluid, to the blood. This makes the lymphatic vessels an auxiliary part of the circulatory system.

The Heart

The heart is a four-chambered muscular organ (Fig. 2–10). Its main responsibility is to pump blood with sufficient pressure to meet the needs of the body's cells and to keep blood circulating in the vessels (Fig. 2–11). The heart is enclosed by the pericardium. It is a tough, white fibrous tissue. It is lined by a double-layer membrane. The inner layer or epicardium forms the outer layer of the heart itself. Beneath the epicardium is the myocardium or the main layer of the heart which is composed of cardiac muscle and forms most of the heart wall. The heart is divided into two parts by this wall. Each part is composed of an upper chamber (atrium) and a lower chamber (ventricle). The right atrium receives deoxygenated blood from various parts of the body primarily through the two veins called the superior vena cava and the inferior vena cava. The superior vena cava brings blood from the body parts superior, or above, to the heart. The inferior vena cava brings blood from the body parts inferior, or below, to the heart. The blood flows from the right atrium to the right ventricle which pumps it to the lungs. Here in the lungs, the blood releases carbon dioxide and picks up oxygen. The oxygenated blood returns to the left atrium in the heart. It then passes to the left ventricle and out of the heart where it is distributed via the aorta, the largest artery, to circulate throughout the body. This pattern of blood flow

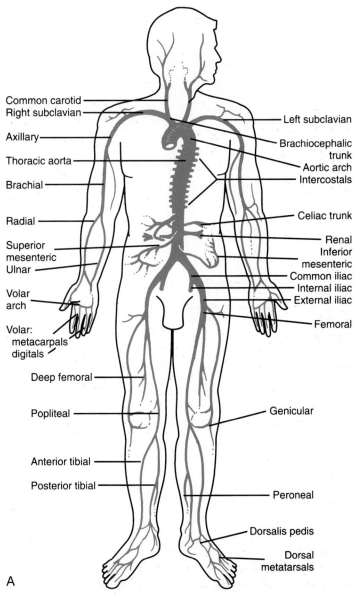

FIGURE 2-9 • Blood Vessels. *A*, The major arteries.

Illustration continued on following page

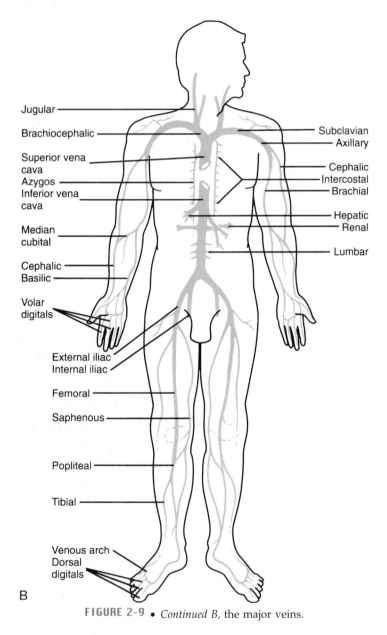

Jugular

Brachiocephalic

Superior vena cava

Azygos

Inferior vena cava

Median cubital

Cephalic

Basilic

Volar digitals

External iliac

Internal iliac

Femoral

Saphenous

Popliteal

Tibial

Venous arch

Dorsal digitals

Subclavian

Axillary

Cephalic

Intercostal

Brachial

Hepatic

Renal

Lumbar

B

FIGURE 2-9 • *Continued B, the major veins.*

is maintained by valves within the heart's chambers which prevent any backflow from ventricles to atrium. The four valves in the heart are the tricuspid, mitrial, pulmonary, and aortic semilunar. A heart murmur is caused when one of the valves does not close properly and blood leaks into it.

Heartbeat and Blood Pressure

The rhythmical nature of cardiac muscle contraction (heartbeat) originates in and through the heart with no extrinsic stimulation. Small masses, or nodes, make up the conductive system in the heart which emits the electrical impulses. The heartbeat originates in the S–A node (sinu–atrial) and is therefore called the "pacemaker" of the heart.

The heart is stimulated by the ANS. These nerves alter the heart rate but are not responsible for the heartbeat. At resting state, the heart beats approximately 70-72 beats per minute. One complete contraction/relaxation cycle lasts about 0.8 second. Exercise, emotions, hormones,

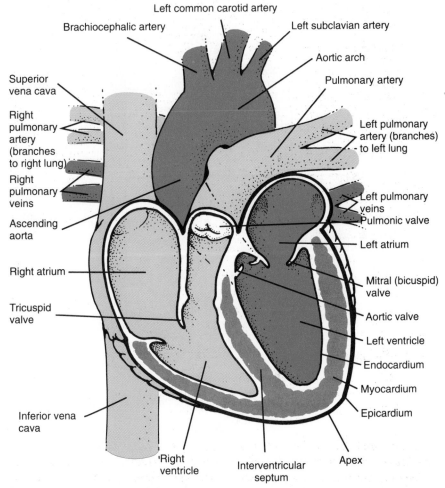

FIGURE 2-10 • Diagram of the heart showing the chambers, valves, and direction of blood flow.

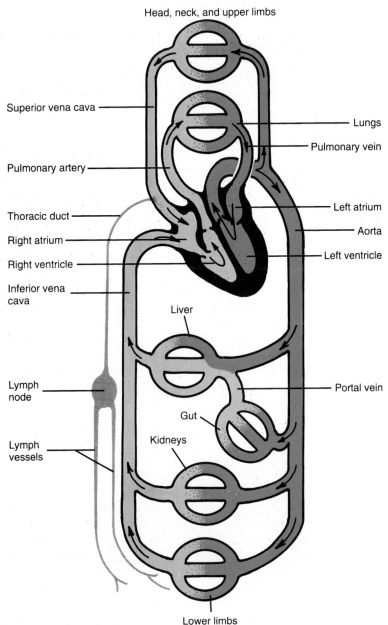

FIGURE 2-11 • The blood circuit.

drugs, and body temperature are some factors that can influence heart rate. The electrocardiogram (ECG or EKG) records electrical potentials generated by the heart. Abnormalities in heart rate can be detected with its use. More details on ECGs are located in Chapter 8.

The cardiac cycle is composed of a phase of contraction **(systole)** and a phase of relaxation **(diastole).** These phases are the basis for the interpretation of blood pressure measurements. Blood pressure is produced by the contraction of the heart muscle. It is defined as the force with which blood pushes against blood vessel walls. It is measured in terms of millimeters of mercury (mm Hg) by using a **sphygmomanometer** or blood pressure cuff. The cuff is placed around the arm and inflated to compress the brachial artery. **(Note:** The leg may also be used. The femoral artery is compressed in this case.) The stethoscope is placed above the bend of the elbow and air pressure in the cuff is released slowly. The first sound heard represents the artery beginning to open. This is recorded as systolic blood pressure. The sounds decrease in intensity until no longer audible as blood freely flows through the vessel. The last audible sound is the diastolic blood pressure. Normal blood pressure varies between individuals but it is usually written as systolic/diastolic or 120/80 mm Hg.

Many factors influence blood pressure. They include total blood volume, thickness of blood, and elasticity and diameter of the blood vessels. Blood pressure is very helpful in the diagnosis of heart diseases such as **coronary heart disease, artherosclerosis,** and **arrhythmias.** High blood pressure **(hypertension)** is associated with a higher risk of a cardiovascular accident (stroke) or a myocardial infarction (heart attack). **Hypotension** or low blood pressure can also cause serious medical problems. The medical specialty that studies the heart is cardiology.

Blood Vessels

There are three kinds of blood vessels (Fig. 2–12):

1. Arteries carry oxygenated blood away from the heart. Exceptions to this include pulmonary and umbilical arteries which carry unoxygenated blood to the lungs and placenta, respectively, for oxygenation (see Fig. 2–11). They are composed of three layers of tissue and have very thick walls. The arterial system branches out from the largest artery, the aorta, to the smallest of the arteries called the arterioles.

2. Capillaries receive the flow of blood from the arteries. Capillaries are very narrow. They are most important to circulation because it is through their walls that all oxygen, nutrients, and waste products pass between the blood and cells.

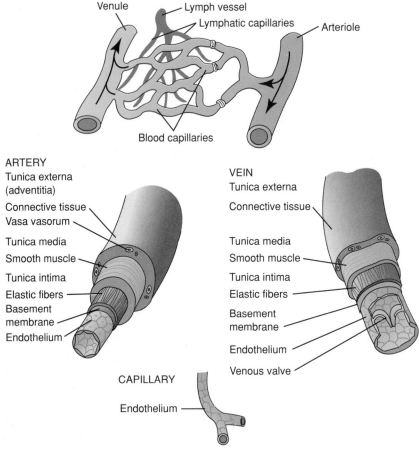

FIGURE 2-12 • Structure of blood vessels and blood flow through them. (Modified with permission from Applegate, EJ: The Anatomy and Physiology Learning System. Philadelphia, PA, WB Saunders, 1995.)

3. Venules receive blood flow from the capillaries. Venules empty blood into larger veins. Pressure in the veins is low so they are equipped with valves to prevent the backflow of blood. The veins carry deoxygenated blood to the heart. Veins are also composed of three layers of tissue but their walls are very fine.

The diameter of the blood vessels can be altered by changes in the walls of the vessels. The vessels can narrow (constrict) or widen (dilate). The changes control blood pressure in the vessels. The pulse is an index of the heart's actions, the elasticity of the vessels, and the resistance in the capillaries and arterioles. Arterial pulse can be taken from the brachial, femoral, and radial arteries. Pulse is evaluated by the following criteria: rate, rhythm, and strength. The normal resting pulse for an adult is 60 to

80 beats per minute. An increase is seen after exercise and in medical conditions associated with fever. It is decreased during sleep.

The Blood

Blood consists of the formed elements (cells and cell fragments) and a liquid component called plasma. Plasma is approximately 90% water. The other 10% consists of plasma proteins, amino acids, hormones, electrolytes, gases, antibodies, and other nutrients. Plasma makes up about 55% of total blood volume. The remaining 45% are the formed elements or cells. The three classes of formed elements are erythrocytes (red blood cells), leukocytes (white blood cells), and thrombocytes (platelets). Fig. 2–13 shows the different types of cells found in the blood.

Red blood cells are biconcave disks which allows them to be flexible when traveling through veins and capillaries. They are the most numerous of the formed elements (Table 2–1). The primary function of the red cells is to carry oxygen in the bloodstream. This is accomplished by the presence of the **hemoglobin** molecule within the cell. Hemoglobin contains iron and gives the red cell its color. Normal erythrocytes live for about 120 days. At the end of their life cycle, they are removed from circulation by the liver or spleen. The iron and protein in the hemoglobin are recycled by the body.

There are two main classifications of white blood cells: granulocytes and agranulocytes. Granulocytes have granules in the cytoplasm while agranulocytes do not. Neutrophils are the most common type of granulocyte (see Table 2–1). They engulf bacteria by **phagocytosis** and are significantly increased in acute infections. They are known as polymorphonuclear leukocytes or segmented neutrophils because their nucleus is multilobed with the average of three to five lobes per cell.

Eosinophils have a bilobed nucleus and large granules that stain red–orange. They increase in allergic reactions or parasitic infections. Basophils are the least common leukocyte. They also have a bilobed nucleus and large granules; however, these granules stain blue–black. They secrete histamine and heparin. Histamine increases blood flow to damaged vessels and heparin acts as an anticoagulant.

The agranulocytes include the lymphocytes and monocytes. Lymphocytes protect the body and provide immunity. They are abundant in the lymphatic system. The T-lymphocytes attack bacteria and viruses while the B-lymphocytes produce antibodies that react with microorganisms or their toxins. Monocytes are the largest white blood cells and they engage in phagocytosis. They can leave the blood and enter the tissues. In the tissue they are called macrophages. They continue the cleansing process within the tissue.

Thrombocytes are cell fragments that aid in blood clotting. When a blood vessel is damaged, platelets adhere to the surface and begin to

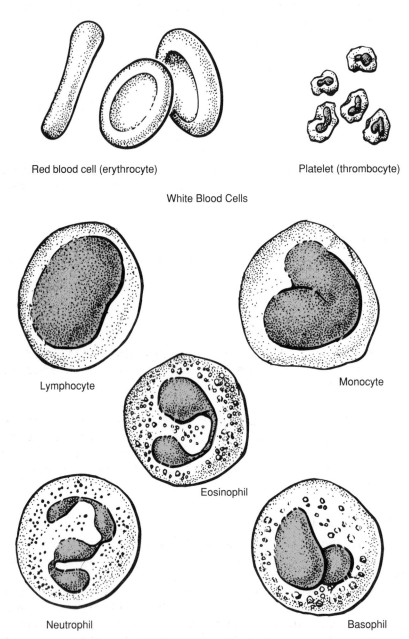

Red blood cell (erythrocyte)

Platelet (thrombocyte)

White Blood Cells

Lymphocyte

Monocyte

Eosinophil

Neutrophil

Basophil

FIGURE 2-13 • Blood cells.

TABLE 2-1 • Normal Blood Cell Values for an Adult

Red blood cells	$4.50-6.00 \times 10^{12}/L$
White blood cells	$4.5-11.0 \times 10^{9}/L$
Neutrophils	45–70%
Lymphocytes	20–40%
Monocytes	3–8%
Eosinophils	2–4%
Basophils	1–2%
Platelets	$150-450 \times 10^{9}/L$

clump or aggregate together so clotting occurs. When not utilized for clotting, platelets remain in circulation nine or ten days before entering the spleen.

Coagulation

The process of coagulation or **hemostasis** involves three steps that result in clot formation preventing excessive blood loss:

1. The damaged blood vessels constrict to reduce flow of blood.

2. A platelet plug is formed.

3. A series of reactions occur in a specified sequence or cascade so that a product of one reaction catalyzes the next. Many factors are necessary for clotting to occur (Fig. 2–14).

The final product of these steps is fibrin which is a meshwork that traps cells and platelets into a clot. (In a test tube, the remaining liquid portion of the blood after a clot is formed is serum.) There is a delicate balance between clot formation and fibrinolysis (dissolving of a clot) within the body to maintain hemostasis.

Blood Typing

If an individual loses a large quantity of blood, it may be necessary to give the person a transfusion of blood, plasma, platelets, or other component to replenish those lost. Serological testing for the transfusion of red blood cells is important to correctly identify blood group **antigens** located on the surface of red blood cells. Commercially prepared antisera **(antibodies)** agglutinate or clump with their corresponding antigens. There are many blood group antigens (Table 2–2); however, ABO and Rh groups are most important. When considering the transfusion of red blood cells, antibodies in the recipient's plasma must also be considered. In the ABO blood group these antibodies are naturally occurring without

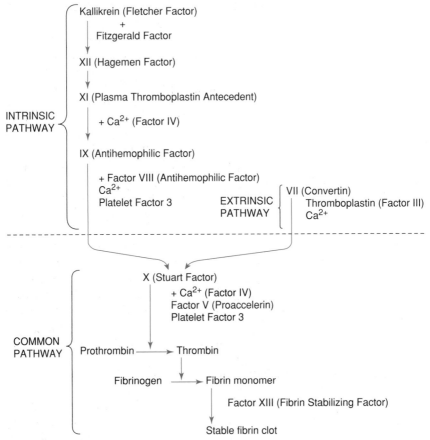

FIGURE 2-14 • Simplified coagulation cascade showing intrinsic, extrinsic, and common pathways.

TABLE 2-2 • Blood Group Systems and Their Common Antigens

Blood Group	Antigens
Rh	D, C, c, E, e
MNS	M, N, S, s
Kell	K, k
Duffy	Fy^a, Fy^b
Kidd	Jk^a, Jk^b
Lewis	Le^a, Le^b

known stimulus, while most other blood group antibody production is stimulated by previous transfusion or pregnancy.

The ABO blood groups are based on the presence or absence of antigens on the cells (Fig. 2–15). Table 2–3 lists the antigens and antibodies for each blood type in the ABO system. Notice that an individual cannot have the same antigen and antibody present. They will produce antibodies to whichever antigen is not present on their own red blood cells.

It is best to give blood of a matching type to avoid adverse reactions called transfusion reactions. A transfusion reaction is caused when a foreign antigen from donor cells reacts with antibodies formed in the recipient. These reactions can range from being mild, causing hives or a slight fever, to severe, resulting in death. In emergencies, an AB type person can receive blood of any ABO type and an O type person can give blood to any ABO type (Table 2–3).

Rh factor, or the D antigen, is the second blood group considered when transfusing blood products. About 85% of the Caucasian population is Rh or D positive and 15% is Rh or D negative and approximately 91% of the African-American population is Rh positive. When transfusions are given, both ABO and Rh type should match between donor and recipient.

The Lymphatic System

The lymphatic system (Fig. 2–16), primarily a system of vessels and tissues nodules, works in conjunction with the circulatory system to carry fluid through the vessels. This system has three main functions within the body. It returns interstitial fluid or fluid from the spaces between cells to the blood from which it came. When this fluid passes from the spaces into the lymphatic vessels, it is called lymph. Lymphatic vessels are similar to veins in structure but have more valves than veins. The vessels join to form the lymphatic trunks that merge until the lymph enters two ducts. The right lymphatic duct collects lymph from the upper right quadrant of the body and empties it into the right subclavian vein. The thoracic duct, the largest lymphatic duct in the body, collects lymph from all other regions of the body and empties it into the left subclavian vein. Lymph nodes are distributed along the vessels at varying intervals. A lymph node is a mass of lymphoid tissue that filters bacteria and other foreign material from the lymph before allowing it to return to circulation.

The second function of the lymphatic system is the collection of fat and fat-soluble vitamins from the digestive process. It transports these via lymph capillaries called lacteals to the general circulation. The lymph in the lacteals is usually milky in appearance because it has such a high fat content.

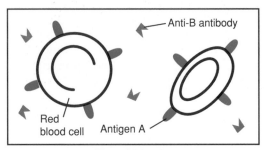

Type A blood

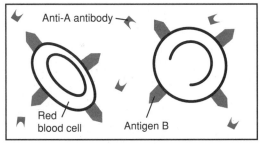

Type B blood

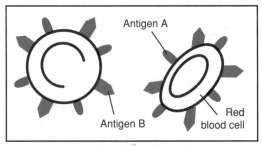

Type AB blood

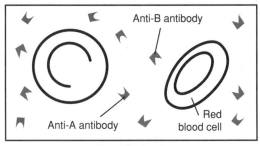

Type O blood

FIGURE 2-15 • Blood groups. Antigens and antibodies in the A, B, AB, and O blood groups.

TABLE 2-3 • The ABO Blood Group System

Blood Type	Antigen	Antibodies	Can Receive From	Can Donate To
A	A	Anti-B	A, O	A, AB
B	B	Anti-A	B, O	B, AB
AB	A, B	None	AB, A, B, O	AB
O	None	Anti-A, anti-B	O	O, A, B, AB

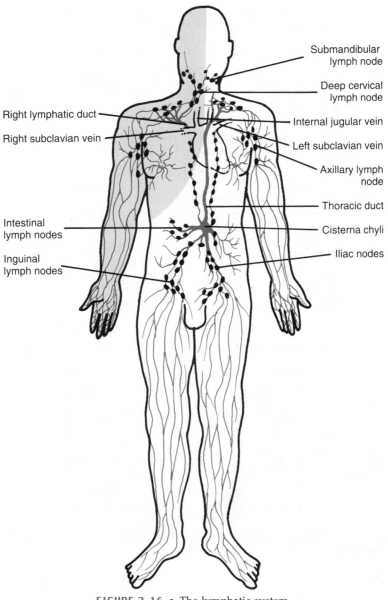

FIGURE 2-16 • The lymphatic system.

The lymphatic system also plays an important role in immunity and defense by providing the body with lymphocytes that fight against infection and disease. These lymphocytes mature in the thymus, one of the lymphatic organs. The spleen and tonsils also serve as part of the lymphatic system. The spleen acts as a filtration system much like the lymph nodes do. Tonsils function to prevent infection by way of nose or mouth.

SYSTEMS INVOLVED IN ENERGY METABOLISM

The Respiratory System

The respiratory system serves the body in three ways: respiration, circulation, and pH maintenance. The respiration process includes (1) the intake of **oxygen** (O_2) by breathing or ventilation into the lungs; (2) the exchange of gases between the lungs and blood; (3) subsequent exchange of gases from the blood to tissue; and (4) the transport of **carbon dioxide** (CO_2) back to the atmosphere. Figure 2–17 shows the path of air flow from the nasal cavity into the lungs.

The lungs are the organs of respiration. The right lung has three lobes and is shorter than the left lung because the liver forces the diaphragm up. It has a greater volume than the left lung, which has only two lobes.

The blood transports the respiratory gases (O_2 and CO_2) between the lungs and tissues. Hemoglobin in the red blood cells has the ability to bind and/or release O_2 as the tissue cells' demand for O_2 increases and

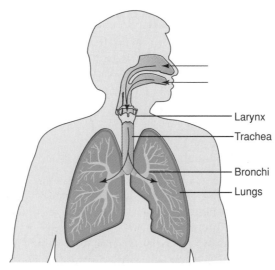

Larynx
Trachea
Bronchi
Lungs

FIGURE 2-17 • The respiratory system showing flow of air into lungs.

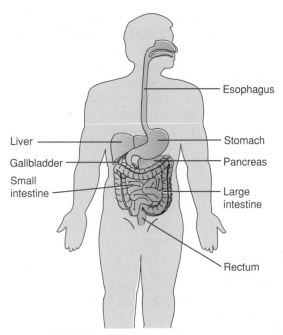

FIGURE 2-18 • The digestive system.

decreases within the body. Factors such as temperature, pH, O_2 levels, and CO_2 levels influence this process. CO_2, a waste product of metabolism, is carried by the blood to the lungs. It can be carried in the plasma or by the hemoglobin molecule and bicarbonate ions within the red blood cells. Because the CO_2 content in the lungs is low, the CO_2 diffuses into the lungs and is exhaled.

The pH of the blood is regulated by the increase and decrease of CO_2. An increase in CO_2 reduces the pH of the blood, which makes the blood more acidic. A decrease in CO_2 increases the pH of the blood, which makes the blood more alkaline. A pulmonologist studies the lungs and related respiratory organs.

The Digestive System

Food must be broken down into small molecules so that it can be digested, absorbed, and metabolized by the body. The digestive system (Fig. 2–18) is responsible for these functions. After food is ingested, chewed, and swallowed, it moves down the esophagus into the stomach. Gastric glands in the stomach secrete gastric juice which is comprised of hydrochloric acid, mucus, enzymes, and other fluids. Food particles mix with these and are then emptied into the small intestine by peristalsis.

Peristalsis is the rhythmic wave of smooth muscle contraction. It is here, in the small intestine, that digestion is completed. Intestinal enzymes and products produced by the liver, gall bladder, and pancreas are required elements to aid in this process. The liver produces bile which is concentrated and stored in the gall bladder until needed. Bile contains bile salts which help in the digestion of fat molecules. The pancreas produces enzymes such as amylase and lipase which help to breakdown complex carbohydrates and fatty acids. Nutrients are then absorbed and the remainder is passed on to the large intestine.

Absorption occurs by active transport across cell membranes through villi that line the inner surface of the small intestine. Each villus contains a blood capillary and a lymphatic capillary (lacteal). Simple sugars and amino acids pass into the blood capillaries while fatty acids enter the lacteals. In the large intestine, water and electrolytes are absorbed and waste products are excreted via the rectum and anus.

After nutrients are absorbed, they are utilized by the body to produce energy for all the chemical reactions that occur. These chemical reactions are called **metabolism.** Metabolic reactions are divided into two categories: anabolism and catabolism. Anabolism is the process of making larger molecules from smaller ones. This requires the use of chemical energy or ATP (adenosine triphosphate). Catabolism is the breakdown of large molecules into smaller ones. Energy is released during catabolism.

The Renal System

Urinary Function

The primary function of the urinary system (Fig. 2–19) is to maintain fluid hemostasis or balance in the body. It consists of a pair of kidneys, ureters, bladder, and urethra.

The kidneys filter the blood to remove waste products and excrete them into the urine. The functional unit in the kidney is called a nephron. Blood flows into the kidney where it is filtered by the glomerulus, a cluster of capillaries, within the nephron. Urine then passes from the nephrons into the bladder via the ureters. The bladder is a temporary storage area for the urine. Urine exits the body through the urethra which is controlled by voluntary skeletal muscle. In men, the urethra, which is much longer than in females, transports both urine and semen. The urethra passes through the prostate gland and penis.

After the filtration process, useful substances and water are moved from the filtrate in the kidney to the blood. This process is called reabsorption. The kidneys alter the concentration and volume of urine. This helps to maintain blood concentration, volume, and pressure. Other

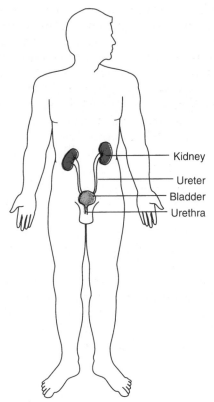

FIGURE 2-19 • The urinary system.

functions of the kidneys include renin and erythropoietin production. Renin is an enzyme that is made in response to a low blood pressure or low sodium concentration. It stimulates vasoconstrictor production to increase blood pressure. Erythropoietin is a hormone that controls red blood cell production in the bone marrow. The study of the urinary system is known as urology.

The Reproductive System

The reproductive system involves mechanisms that work together to produce offspring. The primary reproductive organs, or **gonads,** are the testes in males and the ovaries in females (Fig. 2–20*A* and 2-20*B*). The ovaries produce egg cells, or ova, and the testes produce spermatazoa, or

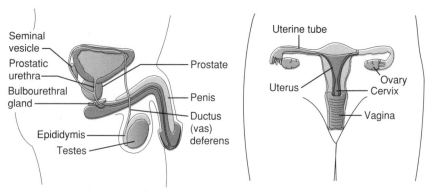

FIGURE 2-20 • *A*, The male and *B*, the female reproductive systems.

sperm cells. These sex cells, or gametes, also produce hormones that are important in the reproductive process. Testosterone, an **androgen,** is necessary for the development and function of the male reproductive organs and for the development and maintenance of secondary male sex characteristics. The primary female hormones are the estrogens. They induce ovulation and the growth of female reproductive structures. Estrogens are also responsible for the development of secondary female sex characteristics. Progesterone and other hormones secreted by the pituitary gland help to regulate the functions of the female reproductive system.

Sperm cell production in the testes begins at the onset of puberty and continues throughout the life of a male. Sperm are released from the testes, enter the epididymis—a series of ducts—where they mature and are stored. They then pass through the urethra and penis where they exit the body. The seminal vesicles, prostate, and bulburethral (Cowper's) glands secrete fluids that form semen. Semen is a mixture of these secretions and sperm.

The female reproductive system includes the ovaries, uterus, vagina, uterine tubes, external genitalia, and glands. The menstrual cycle takes place from the onset of puberty until menopause. During the menstrual cycle, a single mature ovum is released from the ovaries. This is called ovulation. The lining of the uterus prepares for implantation of the egg if it should become fertilized by a sperm.

This process occurs under the influence of hormones whose levels have gradually risen during the cycle. If the egg is not fertilized during ovulation, hormone levels decline and menstruation begins. During the menstrual cycle the ovaries produce estrogen and progesterone that stimulate the development of the uterus's lining, or endometrium. The pituitary hormone production is subsequently inhibited and this cyclic pattern continues. If fertilization occurs, the zygote (fertilized egg) attaches to the wall of the uterus and begins to develop into a fetus.

REVIEW QUESTIONS

1. The _____ is the smallest unit of life.
2. A group of organs working together to perform

   related functions is defined as a _____ .

3. _____ muscle makes up the heart.

4. The _____ are responsible for producing gametes.

5. _____ aid in the coagulation process by
   forming a plug to stop blood flow.
6. The digestion process is completed in the

   _____ .

7. Blood transports the respiratory gases of

   _____ and _____ between the
   lungs and the tissues.

8. The _____ system plays an important
   role in immunity and defense against infection.

9. The _____ alter the concentration and
   volume of urine.
10. The three kinds of blood vessels are

    _____ , _____ , and _____ .

11. A _____ plane divides an organ into
    superior and posterior portions.
12. The skin, one of the largest organs in the body,

    is part of the _____ system.
13. Chemicals used by the body to carry impluses

    between neurons are called _____ .

14. The five types of white blood cells are

_____ , _____ , _____ ,

_____ , and _____ .

15. _____ is released during the process of catabolism.

References

1. Applegate EJ: The Anatomy and Physiology Learning System: Textbook. Philadelphia, WB Saunders, 1995.
2. Ganong WF: Review of Medical Physiology, 16th ed. Norwalk, CT, Appleton & Lange, 1993.
3. Gray H: Gray's Anatomy. NJ, Chartwell Books, 1991.
4. Marleb EN: Human Anatomy & Physiology, 4th ed. CA, The Benjamin/Cummings Publishing Company, 1998.
5. Tortora GL, Anagnostokos NP: Principles of Anatomy and Physiology. 6th ed. New York, Harper and Row Publishers, 1990.

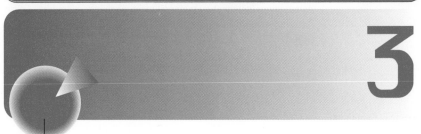

CHAPTER 3

Infectious Diseases and Their Prevention

Georganne K. Buescher

• Infection Control Practices

Isolation Procedures
Antibiotic-Resistant Organisms Precautions
Patient Protection Precautions
Blood Culture Collection and Bacteremia

Numerous diseases can be transmitted by contact with an infected person or a source of contamination. Phlebotomists, as health care professionals, will be asked to take blood from **infectious** persons, and it is therefore important for them to become familiar with the infectious diseases that pose the greatest risk to them. Occupational transmission of bloodborne pathogens has emerged, over the last decade, as one of the most significant hazards to health care workers. The increased awareness of bloodborne pathogens is due primarily to studies demonstrating that the human immunodeficiency virus (HIV) is an occupational hazard to health care workers and the availability of immunization for health care workers to eliminate transmission of the hepatitis B virus.[1] This chapter will familiarize health care workers with those infections that pose occupational risks for phlebotomists and the precautions that must be taken for protection. Many patients with transmissible, blood-borne diseases such as chronic hepatitis (hepatitis B, hepatitis C) or the human immunodeficiency virus (HIV) infection may be asymptomatic when they are admitted to the hospital and unaware that they are infected. In contrast to hepatitis B, there are no vaccines or efficacious postexposure prophylaxis for Hepatitis C or HIV virus. However, the risk of transmission to the phlebotomist is extremely low if proper control and preventive measures are learned and carried out for all patients. Frequent, thorough handwashing (Table 3–1) is the single most important preventive measure to reduce the risks of transmitting organisms from one person to another,

---

TABLE 3-1 • Acceptable Hand Washing Technique

1. Wash hands before and after entering a patient's room.
2. Remove jewelry on hands and wrists.
3. Wet hands under running water.
4. Keep hands down and apply soap or antiseptic hand scrub.
5. Employ friction to clean all surfaces of the hands and wrists.
6. Rinse thoroughly under running water.
7. Dry hands thoroughly with paper towels.
8. Use paper towels to turn off the faucet to prevent contamination.

from one location to another, and from one anatomical site on the same patient to another site.

Pathogens of all four major groups of microorganisms (bacteria, fungi, viruses, and parasites) may be carried in the blood during the course of a specific disease. Over the years, the risk of occupation-associated infections has shifted in focus from bacterial to viral infections. Today, percutaneously transmitted pathogens of greatest concern to health care professionals can be limited to bloodborne, viral infections; hepatitis B virus; hepatitis C virus; and HIV.

VIRAL INFECTIOUS DISEASES

Viral **nosocomial** infections are an important **epidemiologic** concern for health care providers. Studies have shown patterns in the transmission of bloodborne pathogens that implicate serum viral concentrations and the dose of an exposure as the critical factors for transmission. Because of their contact with patients, phlebotomists are at risk for transmission of vaccine-preventable viral diseases. Immunization protocols for employees in health care institutions can provide safeguards against infection for personnel as well as for patients, since viruses can be transmitted from patients to staff, as well as from staff to patients.

Today there is a focus on the health care institution's responsibility to protect employees from infection. The institution must ensure that employees such as phlebotomists who are at risk for infection have been immunized properly. Laboratory screening tests are available to determine a person's immunization status for a wide range of infectious diseases, including hepatitis, measles, polio, mumps, rubella, and chickenpox.

Over the last decade several trends have emerged in the transmission of viral infections. Both HIV and hepatitis B virus infections have increased in prevalence among hospitalized patients. Evidence suggests that while the prevalence of hepatitis B virus has increased among patients, the incidence of hepatitis B among health care professionals has decreased as a result of immunization of personnel with the hepatitis B vaccine. Prevalence studies of hepatitis C virus among patients show that the number of cases is even higher than that of hepatitis B and HIV. Unlike hepatitis B, there are no vaccines or efficacious postexposure prophylaxis for hepatitis C and HIV virus, so we are forced to rely on other control and preventive measures to reduce transmission.

percutaneous

VIRAL HEPATITIS

Hepatitis is a systemic disease primarily involving the liver. There are several types of hepatitis virus infections with differing modes of

TABLE 3-2 • Characteristics of Acute Viral Hepatitis

	Hepatitis A (HAV)	Hepatitis B (HBV)	Hepatitis C (HCV)
Epidemiology	Fecal-oral	Parenteral	Parenteral and nonparenteral
Incubation period (days)	15–45	40–180	15–150
Asymptomatic infection	Usual	Common	Common
Chronicity	No	Yes	Yes

transmission: hepatitis A virus (HAV), also known as infectious hepatitis or short incubation hepatitis; HBV, also known as serum hepatitis or long-incubation hepatitis; and hepatitis C virus (HCV), which is associated with chronic viral hepatitis. All types of viral hepatitis produce an acute inflammation of the liver, which causes a clinical illness characterized by fever, nausea, vomiting, and jaundice. Table 3–2 presents a comparison of HAV, HBV, and HCV infections.

HAV is transmitted most often by the fecal-oral route. Phlebotomists may become infected by contact with a patient's feces or blood.

HCV transmission pattern, since screening test have become available, has shifted from contaminated blood to the sharing of contaminated needles used for "recreational" drug delivery.

HBV Infection

HBV infection is recognized by the Centers for Disease Control and Prevention (CDC) as a major occupational hazard for health care workers. It is the most frequently reported occupation-associated infection for persons who handle blood or blood products. The risk of infection is much higher for health care professionals than for the general population, and worldwide, HBV is a leading cause of acute and chronic hepatitis, cirrhosis of the liver, and primary hepatocellular carcinoma. Phlebotomists, because of the procedures that they perform, are at risk for HBV infection from needlesticks with contaminated needles.

HBV is global in its distribution. Chronic carriers may or may not have the typical signs and symptoms of liver disease and may not be recognized as high-risk patients (i.e., patients with infections that can be passed on to those who care for them).

The incubation period for HBV is between 50 and 180 days, with a mean onset time of 60 to 90 days after transmission.

Prevention

The risk of acquiring HBV infection from occupational exposures depends on the frequency of percutaneous or **permucosal** exposures to blood or blood products. As little as 0.0001 ml of infected **plasma** (about 1/500 of a drop—much too small to see) can transmit this disease. Therefore, an important preventive measure to reduce the potential for HBV transmission is the use of gloves.

HBV is a vaccine-preventable disease, and therefore Federal Occupational Safety and Health Administration (OSHA) regulations require that all health care personnel at risk for exposure to HBV receive hepatitis B vaccination. A blood test can be done to be sure protective antibodies have developed. A consistent program of vaccinations would eliminate the problem of having susceptible health care workers in hospitals.[2]

The CDC has developed guidelines for efficacious postexposure **prophylaxis** in a nonimmune individual exposed to HBV.

Patients with an acute HBV infection generally are not placed in strict isolation when they are hospitalized. They may remain in a regular room as long as blood and instrument precautions are strictly followed on the floor and in the laboratory.

HCV INFECTION

Hepatitis C (HCV) is an RNA virus of the *Flaviviridae* family. This genetically diverse virus has at least six genotypes and numerous serotypes. It is this diversity that is thought to enable HCV to escape the host's immune surveillance, leading to an 85% rate of infected individuals who become chronic carriers. The CDC estimates the number of individuals in the United States infected with HCV at 4 million. There are 30,000 new infections each year, an estimated 8,000 deaths annually and, without an available vaccine, the number of new cases is predicted to triple over the next 15–20 years. More than 20% of the patients with chronic HCV infections develop cirrhosis, making HCV now the leading reason for liver transplantation.

HCV infection can lead to acute and chronic infections which can lead to cirrhosis, liver cancer or failure, and death.

A variety of tests are now available for diagnosing HCV infection which detect HCV or its components: enzyme immunoassay (EIA), a recombinant immunoblot assay, several PCR-based tests. Typically, the diagnosis is made with EIA and liver enzyme function tests.

Health care professionals have a higher prevalence of infection which provides some evidence of occupational nosocomial transmission. While infection may have been acquired outside of the work environment, needlestick injuries and a lapse in the application of universal precautions may be contributing factors. Studies have shown that the risk of infection with HCV is between that of HIV and HBV.[3]

Prevention

Although HCV is the leading cause of chronic viral hepatitis in the U.S., the development of an effective vaccine has been hindered by its extensive genetic diversity. Adherence to universal precautions for the protection of health care professionals and patients is essential to avoid transmission of hepatitis C.

Alpha-interferon is the standard course of therapy for HCV infection, although it does not lead to complete clearance of the virus even after twelve months of therapy. Patients are also urged to abstain from alcohol and to be vaccinated against HBV and HAV. A combination therapy of interferon and ribavirin is being used in clinical trials for patients who relapsed.[4]

HIV INFECTION

HIV is a member of the retrovirus family of RNA viruses. It is the primary etiologic agent of the acquired immunodeficiency syndrome (AIDS) and the AIDS-related complex. AIDS was first described in 1981, but it was not until 1983 that the causative viral agent was isolated. Today, AIDS has reached epidemic proportions worldwide, with tens of thousands of cases in the United States.

After transmission of HIV, a high percentage of infected carriers will go on to develop a fatal illness. The virus replicates slowly but continuously, generally taking several years before it begins to attack and destroy the person's T-helper lymphocytes and macrophages. The destruction of these cells leads to deficiencies in multiple branches of the person's immune system. The incubation period for adults is between 6 months and 7 years. To date, the male homosexual population has the highest rate of infection in the United States. Other populations at high risk for infection include bisexual males, intravenous drug abusers, hemophiliacs who received contaminated blood products before 1985, and male or female sexual partners of persons in any of the previous groups. Pediatric AIDS cases differ from those in adults in that neonates acquire the infection from mothers who are infected. The onset of symptoms in such children generally occurs by the age of 2.

AIDS is not a single disease, but rather a collection of various diseases that characteristically develop in patients who are HIV positive. The HIV virus suppresses the immune system, making the patient susceptible to unusual neoplasms such as Kaposi's sarcoma, a wide variety of severe opportunistic infections, and neurologic disorders. The diagnosis of HIV infection in asymptomatic patients is made by testing for specific antibodies formed against the virus or by detecting the virus. Serologic tests in persons who have been infected with the HIV generally become positive within 2 months of exposure to the virus. It is very uncommon for an infected person to go more than 6 months without a detectable antibody response.

Since 1983, there have been several reported cases of transmission of the HIV to health care professionals; the majority of these followed a needlestick injury with contaminated blood. When compared with the total number of needlestick injuries reported by health care professionals, the number of HIV infections is low. It should be remembered that gloves provide protection against spillage and contamination only; they cannot protect the wearer from needlestick injury. However, gloves do protect phlebotomists when they have cuts, scratches, or other breaks in the skin.

Health care professionals caring for AIDS patients should be familiar with the types of infections seen in these patients so that appropriate protective measures can be employed when needed. The most common severe infectious complications of AIDS include infection with *Pneumocystis carinii* or *Toxoplasma gondii* organisms, *Mycobacterium avium* complex, infection with *Mycobacterium tuberculosis* organisms, cytomegalovirus, herpes simplex virus, HBV, and infection with *Salmonella* or *Cryptococcus* organisms.

Prevention

To date, no vaccine for AIDS has been developed, nor has a therapeutic cure been found. Most exposures do not result in infection. Factors effecting the risk of infection include the type of exposure and (1) the amount of blood involved, (2) the amount of virus in the patient's blood at the time, and (3) whether postexposure treatment was given. Preventive measures rely on the practice of infection control procedures as established by the CDC to prevent transmission of HIV infection to health care professionals. These guidelines, published in 1987, are known as the "Universal Blood and Body-Fluid Precautions,"[4] and are briefly outlined in Table 3–3. The CDC advises that health care organizations operate under the assumption that all patients are potentially infectious. The CDC recommendations state that all health care workers should routinely use **barrier precautions** (i.e., gloves) whenever they are going to be in contact with blood, body fluids, mucous membranes, or the nonintact skin of a patient. A germicidal soap should be used to wash contaminated skin surfaces, and in the event of a spill, the environmental surfaces should be cleansed and decontaminated with a 1:10 dilution of household bleach.

Needlestick protection protocols have also been developed by the CDC to prevent the transmission of infection. Most accidental needlestick injuries occur while attempting to recap a used needle. The protocols

---

TABLE 3-3 • The CDC's Universal Blood and Body Fluid Precautions: A Brief Outline

The Universal Blood and Body Fluid Precautions were designed to prevent parenteral, mucous membrane, and nonintact skin exposure to pathogens among health care practitioners. These guidelines are intended to supplement, not supplant, other recommendations for routine infection control practices. Briefly, the Universal Precautions are as follows:

Infectious fluids are defined as blood, blood products, semen and vaginal secretions, cerebrospinal fluid, synovial fluid, pleural fluid, peritoneal fluid, pericardial fluid, and amniotic fluid

Noninfectious fluids are defined as feces, nasal secretions, sputum, sweat, tears, urine, and vomit (unless blood is present)

Do not recap needles by hand; do not bend or manipulate used needles by hand

Exercise extra caution when using or cleaning any sharp instrument, such as needles, or other laboratory device

Dispose of all sharp items in puncture-resistant waste containers

Use protective barriers such as gloves, gowns, goggles, shields, and masks to prevent exposure to blood and other possibly infectious fluids and materials

Wash skin surfaces immediately and thoroughly after any exposure to an infectious fluid

From Centers for Disease Control (1987). Recommendations for prevention of HIV transmission in health care settings, *MMWR*, 36(suppl 2) 15–185.

---

therefore state that needles should not be recapped, but should be placed in puncture-proof containers that allow for disposal of the needle and syringe without having to recap or cut off the needle.

As the incidence of HIV-positive patients increases, so will the potential for transmission to health care professionals. Education and the

---

▼ What Should Be Done After an Exposure to HIV

- Obtain a base-line test for HIV antibody and at 6 weeks, 12 weeks, and 6 months.
- Postexposure treatment with antiviral drugs with checks for drug toxicity.
- Report any sudden or severe illness with symptoms that may suggest HIV infection, drug reaction, or other medical condition.
- Contact health care provider if there are concerns or problems during the follow-up period.

use of protective measures are the keys to preventing exposure to AIDS and other infectious diseases.

In June 1996 the recommendation of the Public Health Service for postexposure treatment was zidovudine (ZDV), lamivudine (3TC), and the protease inhibitor indinavir (IDV). Treatment should be started preferably within 1–2 hours postexposure. A 4-week course of therapy with ZDV appears to provide protection against HIV infection.[5]

OTHER VIRAL INFECTIOUS DISEASES

Influenza

READ AT HOME

Influenza virus A produces the most serious form of influenza, with symptoms of fever, chills, headache, myalgia, sore throat, and cough. The onset of symptoms is approximately 1 to 4 days after contact with infected respiratory secretions. Infected persons shed the virus for 24 hours before the onset of symptoms and for 3 to 4 days during the course of the disease. Death associated with this virus is usually the result of primary influenza pneumonia or a secondary bacterial pneumonia. The influenza viruses that are the cause of epidemics and nosocomial outbreaks change from season to season, and a new vaccine is manufactured each year.

Prevention

Vaccination, or a "flu shot," is recommended yearly for all health care personnel who have patient contact. Such a program will lower the risk of transmission of influenza from caregivers to patients and reduce the possibility of employee illness and absenteeism because of this virus.[2]

Rubella (German Measles)

Rubella, or German measles, generally produces only a mild illness in children and adults, but can cause congenital malformations if a woman is infected early in her pregnancy. Infection of the fetus can cause severe abnormalities, premature birth, or fetal death. Health care professionals are often young women, and the susceptibility rate in this age group is approximately 10% to 25%. In addition, the risk of contact between an infected professional and pregnant patients is ever present.

Transmission of rubella is from person to person by direct contact with infected respiratory secretions. There is a 2- to 3-week incubation period before symptoms are evident, but the virus begins to be shed from the throat of the patient during the first week after transmission.

PREMARITAL = (M)RPR = SYPHILLIS   WAS A LAW
BLD TEST   (F) RPR + RUBELLA

Prevention

There is no specific antiviral treatment for rubella infection. Vaccination is recommended for all health care professionals who have no proof of previous vaccination or laboratory evidence of immunity.[2] Immunity is long lasting.

Mumps and Measles   *READ AT HOME.*

Mumps is typically not a serious disease, but in a small percentage of cases, complications may be fatal. The most typical symptom is swelling of the parotid salivary glands. The virus is shed in the saliva during the 14- to 24-day incubation period and for about 9 days after the onset of symptoms.

Measles is a systemic infection that often causes a serious illness with pneumonia and secondary bacterial infections. Central nervous system involvement is present in many cases. Teens and young adults account for the majority of cases today. Illness begins with fever, cough, runny nose, and **conjunctivitis** and is characterized by a **maculopapular** rash and bright red spots with a central whitish dot (Koplik's spots) that develop inside the mouth. The measles virus multiplies in the respiratory tract, and infection is transmitted by respiratory secretions. Infected persons are most contagious during the incubation period and the early symptomatic period.

Prevention

Measles and mumps transmission in health care institutions can be disruptive and costly. To prevent such infections, the CDC recommends that all new personnel born in 1957 or later who have direct patient contact should be vaccinated. The measles-mumps-rubella vaccine (MMR) is the vaccine of choice. Persons born before 1957 are considered to be immune to both measles and mumps, because virtually everyone born before that time became infected naturally before the vaccine became available.[2]

Poliovirus   *READ AT HOME!!*

The poliovirus, like other enteroviruses, is transmitted by the fecal-oral route or by respiratory secretions. Most persons infected with this virus are asymptomatic or experience only a mild illness. Poliovirus is shed in the feces for several weeks, and therefore, human feces are the source of virus in the environment. Respiratory shedding of the virus from the throat can last as long as 3 to 4 weeks. Polio is rare in countries such as the United States, and infection is generally limited to nonimmunized persons.

Prevention

There is no specific antiviral therapy for enteroviral infections such as polio. Effective poliovirus vaccines have been available since 1955, when the inactivated vaccine was released, and in 1962, the oral live **attenuated** vaccine was developed. Although live vaccine is less expensive and easier to administer, the virus multiplies, is shed in the feces, and represents a potential risk for transmission to others. Normally the poliovirus vaccine is not routinely recommended for persons older than 18 years. However, the CDC recommends that hospital personnel caring for patients who may be excreting wild polioviruses complete a primary series of poliovirus vaccine.[2]

SELECTED BACTERIAL INFECTIOUS DISEASES

DISEASES CAUSED BY MYCOBACTERIA

Tuberculosis

Both normal individuals and immunocompromised patients (e.g., AIDS patients) may become infected with *M. tuberculosis*, the organism that causes tuberculosis. Tuberculosis is a chronic disease that most frequently produces lesions in the lungs, although disease may develop in other parts of the body. Infection normally occurs by the respiratory route. Patients with this disease are placed under AFB isolation precautions for the protection of the staff and visitors. Antituberculosis drug-resistant strains of *Mycobacterium tuberculosis* are reported. Successful treatment for patients infected with this strain may be problematic, requiring the use of multiple drugs.

Mycobacterium Avium Complex

AIDS patients frequently develop *M. avium* complex infection, which results in high numbers of organisms present in their blood and stool. Infection with these atypical mycobacteria causes AIDS patients to have bouts of diarrhea, as well as respiratory symptoms. Treatment of infection is extremely difficult, requiring multiple drug use because of the organism's high resistance to antituberculosis drugs.

Prevention

Depending on the species of mycobacteria involved in an infection, respiratory precautions (i.e., the use of a respirator) as well as enteric precautions may be required. Antimycobacterial drugs are available and are effective in almost all cases except for the strains mentioned that have developed extreme drug resistance. Administrative controls assume a greater prominence in a TB control program due to the need for early identification, isolation, and treatment of infectious TB patients. OSHA specifically requires that a health care facility do three things for health care workers: (1) offer TB skin tests at no cost to all current employees with potential exposure and to all new employees before exposure, (2) TB skin test at a specified time period determined by risk categories, and (3) provide for employee reassessment following exposure to TB or change in health.[6]

In situations where there is a high risk of exposure to TB (entering rooms housing suspected/confirmed TB cases) OSHA specifically requires that health professionals wear NIOSH-approved respirators. NIOSH issued new criteria, on June 8, 1995, for respirators that would meet the performance criteria set forth by CDC for the prevention of TB. The N-series, those designed for nonoil aerosols, are the ones of most interest for preventing the transmission of TB. In keeping with the guideline requirements, the respirator must be able to (1) filter particles 1 micron in size at an efficiency of ≥95% and at a low of up to 50 liters per minute (L/min), as certified by NIOSH, (2) be reliably fit-tested with a face-seal leakage of ≤10%, (3) fit different-size faces (at least 3), and (4) be checked for facepiece fit by a health professional before every use.[7]

All health care workers, regardless of whether they are at risk of exposure to TB, must receive general training about issues related to tuberculosis before their initial work assignment.

INFECTION BY *SALMONELLA*, *SHIGELLA*, *E. COLI* 0157:H7 AND *CAMPYLOBACTER* SPECIES

Salmonella, Shigella, E. coli 0157:H7 and *Campylobacter* organisms characteristically cause diarrheal diseases. These infections are generally acquired by the oral-fecal route, being transmitted from person to person or in contaminated food or drink. Infected patients are placed on enteric precautions (i.e., the use of gloves and protective clothing), and infected employees are not permitted to have contact with patients or may be sent home until they have tested negative for these organisms. Typhoid fever is caused by one of the species of *Salmonella* and, as may be true for all of these bacteria, may persist in patients, who then become asymptomatic carriers. The feces of asymptomatic carriers are a more important source of contamination than the oral route in symptomatic patients placed on enteric precautions.

E. coli 0157:H7 is the most common cause of enterohemorrhagic *Escherichia coli* (EHEC) characterized by bloody diarrhea, abdominal pain, and an association with the consumption of contaminated food (undercooked beef, unpasteurized cow's milk and apple juice). In approximately 10% of cases, hemolytic uremic syndrome (HUS) will develop characterized by thrombocytopenia, microangiopathic hemolytic anemia, and acute renal failure. This occurs most often in children.

Prevention

Transmission of these organisms is most often by contact with the contaminated hands of health care personnel caring for an infected patient. Thorough hand washing before and after caring for patients is the most effective preventive measure. Effective antibiotic therapy is available for these infections, if necessary.

STAPHYLOCOCCAL INFECTION

The most pathogenic staphylococcus is *Staphylococcus aureus*, which characteristically causes localized abscess formation. *S. aureus* and *Staphylococcus epidermidis* are the most commonly isolated species in health care institutions. Both species are known to develop rapid antibacterial drug resistance. Infections with these strains are increasing in number, and hospitals are experiencing greater difficulty in treating patients with such infections. Contact spread of infection is an important consideration in hospitals, where large proportions of the staff and patients carry antibiotic-resistant *Staphylococcus* organisms in their noses or on their skin. The areas of the hospital where patients are at highest risk for severe staphylococcal infections are the newborn nursery, intensive care units, operating rooms, and chemotherapy units.

Prevention

Patients infected with staphylococci are placed under drainage and secretion precautions. Health care workers are thus alerted to the need for thorough hand-washing practices, as well as the use of gloves when in contact with areas of the patient's body. Staphylococci can be transmitted from contaminated linens and other objects in the environment, as well as directly from abscess secretions. Care should be used in placing equipment or transport devices on surfaces in the room that might contaminate them and thus spread the organism to the next room visited by the caregiver.

INFECTION BY MULTIDRUG RESISTANT ORGANISMS

Increasing incidence of high-level enterococcal resistance to penicillin and aminoglycosides has coincided with vancomycin resistance in enterococci and represents a therapeutic challenge when patients are infected with these microorganisms. The prevention and control of vancomycin resistance requires a comprehensive, institution-specific plan to detect, prevent, and control infection and colonization with VRE.

The potential emergence of vancomycin resistance in clinical isolates of *Staphylococcus aureus* and *Staphylococcus epidermidis* is a great public health concern. The vanA gene, which confers high-level resistance to vancomycin, can be transferred from enterococci to a variety of gram-positive microorganisms.[8]

While there is little or no risks to the phlebotomist of bloodborne transmission of VRE, educational programs for the staff and isolation precautions for the patients are essential to prevent patient-to-patient transmission of this dangerous isolate.

INFECTION CONTROL PRACTICES

ISOLATION PROCEDURES

Isolation procedures were designed to prevent the transmission of infectious agents from patients to personnel or visitors and from personnel or visitors to patients. Personnel and visitors are made aware of the need for special precautions by signs placed outside the patient's room (Fig. 3–1). The precautions recommended for use in health care institutions depend both on the type of infection and on the patient's immunologic status. Infectious agents may be transmitted to patients via the airborne route or may be introduced by contaminated equipment or improper site preparation (as for venipuncture) or site selection. The risk of patient infection from venipuncture or capillary collection is low, although local site infections, as well as more serious infections such as bacteremia, have been associated with these procedures.

Early in 1996, the Centers for Disease Control and Prevention (CDC) and the Hospital Infection Control Practices Advisory Committee (HICPAC) revised the **Recommendations for Isolation Precautions in Hospitals.** New pathogens and multidrug-resistant microorganisms were emerging and yet some health care institutions failed to recognize them as new problems and did not add appropriate precautions for their containment. Clearly what was needed was a new synthesis of the various systems that would provide a guideline with logistically feasible recommendations for preventing the many infections that occur in hospitals

PATIENT CARE

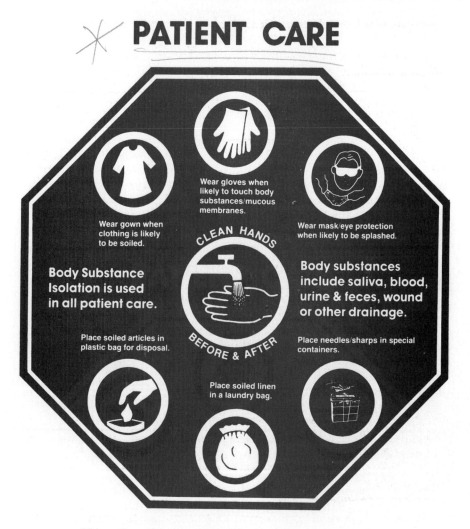

Wear gloves when likely to touch body substances/mucous membranes.

Wear gown when clothing is likely to be soiled.

Wear mask/eye protection when likely to be splashed.

CLEAN HANDS

Body Substance Isolation is used in all patient care.

Body substances include saliva, blood, urine & feces, wound or other drainage.

Place soiled articles in plastic bag for disposal.

BEFORE & AFTER

Place needles/sharps in special containers.

Place soiled linen in a laundry bag.

Body Substance Isolation

FIGURE 3-1 • Sample isolation precaution sign. (Courtesy of Harborview Medical Center, Seattle, WA)

through diverse modes of transmission. For their own protection, phlebotomists must become familiar with the various types of isolation precautions (Table 3–4). The revised recommendations contain three important changes from previous recommendations: (1) **Standard precautions** which synthesized the major features of universal precautions and body substance isolation, (2) the former categories of isolation precautions and disease-specific precautions were collapsed into three sets of precautions based on routes of transmission. Transmission-based precautions were designed to reduce the risk of airborne, droplet, and

---

TABLE 3-4 • New Isolation Categories and Diseases Requiring Specific Isolation Precautions

---

- **Strict Isolation:** Varicella, *Herpes zoster, S. aureus* or *S. pyogenes* (Group A) pneumonia and wounds with uncontrolled drainage. Ebola, Marburg virus and other hemorrhagic viral fevers. Lassa fever, Rabies, Diphtheria, and disseminated Vaccinia virus infection.
- **Contact Isolation:** Acute respiratory infections in infants and children; colds, pharyngitis, croup, bronchitis, epiglottitis, bronchiolitis, and pneumonia until etiology determined—only adenovirus, respiratory syncytial virus, influenza, parainfluenza infections should continue on isolation. Neonatal *Herpes simplex* infection and congenital rubella infections. After 24 hours of effective therapy, isolation may be discontinued for Group A Streptococcal pharyngitis and impetigo.
- **Respiratory Isolation:** Measles, mumps, pertussis, rubella, parvovirus infection. Prior to 24 hours of effective therapy, pneumonia, epiglottitis or meningitis due to *Neisseria meningitidis* or *Haemophilis influenzae* and meningococcemia.
- **AFB Isolation:** Pulmonary and laryngeal tuberculosis
- **Enteric Precautions:** Acute gastroenteritis/diarrheal infections until etiology determined. Enteric Precautions continued for *Shigella* sp., Rotavirus, *E. coli* 0157:H7, *Clostridium difficile*, and acute Hepatitis A virus infections.
- **Resterilization Precautions:** Creutzfield–Jakob disease, Kuru, Gerstmann–Strussler–Scheinker syndrome.
- **Antibiotic-Resistant Organisms Precautions:** Methicillin-resistant *S. aureus* (MRSA), Vancomycin-resistant Enterococci (VRE), Penicillin-resistant *S. pneumoniae*, pan aminoglycoside-resistant Enterobacteriaceae.

Note: Microorganisms/diseases not listed above are to be handled as standard/universal precautions.

contact transmission in hospitals, and are to be used in addition to standard precautions. (3) Specific syndromes in adults and pediatric patients are listed that are highly suspicious for infection and appropriate transmission-based precautions to use on an empiric, temporary basis until a diagnosis can be made or identified.

Standard precautions apply to (1) blood, (2) all body fluid secretions and excretions except sweat, regardless of whether they contain visible blood, (3) nonintact skin, and (4) mucous membranes. Under standard precautions, the following procedures must be observed with all patients:

- **Handwashing and Gloving.** Wear gloves when touching blood, body fluids, secretions, excretions, and contaminated items. Remove gloves promptly after use, before touching noncontaminated items and environmental surfaces. Wash hands immediately after gloves are removed and between patient contacts to avoid transfer of microorganisms to other patients or environment. See Figures 3–2 through 3–6.

- **Mask, Eye Protection, Face Shield.** Wear a mask and eye protection or face shield during procedures and patient-care activities that are likely to generate splashes or sprays of blood, body fluids, secretions, and excretions.

- **Gown.** Wear a gown to protect skin and prevent soiling of clothing during procedures and patient-care activities that are likely to generate splashes or sprays of blood, body fluids, secretions, and excretions, or causes soiling of clothing. Remove a soiled gown as promptly as possible and wash hands to avoid transfer of microorganisms to other patients or environments.

- **Patient-Care Equipment.** Take care to prevent injuries when using needles and when disposing of used needles. Never recap used needles or otherwise manipulate them using both hands, or any other technique that involves directing the point of a needle toward any part of the body. Use either a one-handed "scoop"

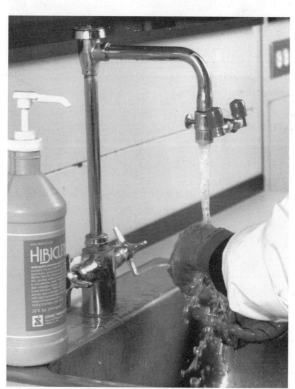

FIGURE 3-2 • Wet hands with warm water. All jewelry should be removed.

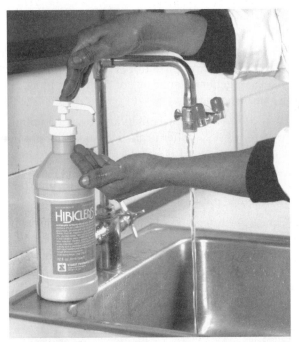

FIGURE 3-3 • Use a generous portion of soap.

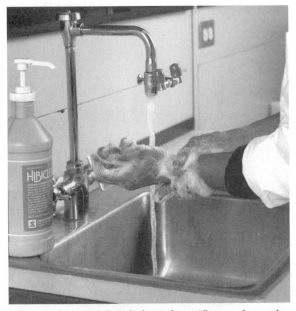

FIGURE 3-4 • Thoroughly scrub hands for at least 15 seconds, work up a lather. Be sure to clean between fingers and wrist.

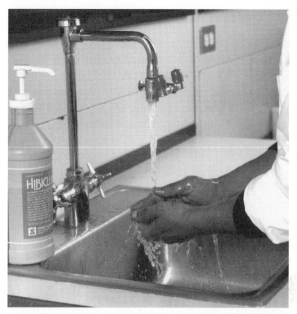

FIGURE 3-5 • Completely rinse hands under warm water. Keep hands in downward position.

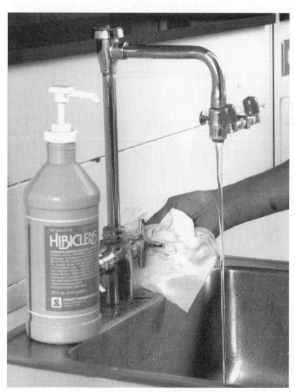

FIGURE 3-6 • Thoroughly dry hands and use a paper towel to turn water off.

technique or a mechanical device designed for holding the needle from disposable syringes by hand. Do not bend, break, or otherwise manipulate used needles by hand. Place used disposable syringes and needles in appropriate puncture-resistant containers located as close as practical in the area in which the items were used. Handle used equipment soiled with blood, body fluid, secretions, and excretions in a manner that prevents skin and mucous membrane exposures, contamination of clothing, and transfer of microorganisms to other patients and environments. Ensure that reusable equipment is not used for the care of another patient until it has been appropriately cleaned and reprocessed and single-use items are properly discarded.

- **Environmental Control.** Ensure that the hospital has adequate procedures for the routine care, cleaning, and disinfection of environmental surfaces, beds, bed-rails, bedside equipment and other frequently touched surfaces and that these procedures are being followed.

- **Linen and Laundry.** Handle transport, and process used linen soiled with blood, body fluids, secretions, and excretions in a manner that prevents skin and mucous membrane exposures, contamination of clothing, and avoid transfer of microorganisms to other patients and environment.

- **Patient Placement.** Place a patient who contaminates the environment or cannot assist in maintaining appropriate hygiene or environmental control in a single room.

Transmission-based precautions should be used as necessary for patients with known infectious diseases such as tuberculosis, influenza, and multi-drug resistant bacteria.

ANTIBIOTIC-RESISTANT ORGANISMS PRECAUTIONS

Patients colonized or infected with methicillin-resistant *S. aureus* (MRSA), vancomycin resistant enterococci (VRE), penicillin-resistant *S. pneumoniae* (PRP), and panaminoglycoside-resistant Enterobacteriaceae are to be placed in a single room and the continuous use of gloves is mandated for health care professionals while in the room. Gloves must be changed when soiled or when changing tasks. Disinfection of all equipment leaving the room is required.

Training in preventive measures will increase the confidence of professionals who care for infected patients. It is the responsibility of the health care institution to conduct inservice education programs in this area for personnel.

PATIENT PROTECTION PRECAUTIONS

A discussion of infection control is not complete unless consideration is given to those groups of patients who are at high risk of infection. Already compromised patients must be protected from infectious agents that might be transmitted by the phlebotomist. The most common high-risk patient areas or groups of patients are discussed below.

Nursery Units. Newborns do not have a fully developed immune system, and thus even healthy infants are at risk of infection. All persons intending to enter the nursery, including phlebotomists, must first wash their hands thoroughly and put on a gown, mask, and gloves. Only the equipment needed to perform the procedure should be taken into the nursery.

The protocol for gowning is as follows: A clean gown is put on with the opening in the back, and then both the neck strings and those at the waist are tied (Table 3–5). If a mask is required, it should be tied high on the head and also behind the head to prevent it from slipping. Gloves are the last barrier protection to be put on and should be pulled on so that the ends fit over the sleeves of the gown. (Table 3–6). After the patient procedure has been completed, the phlebotomist should leave the unit, remove all protective clothing, and dispose of it in the receptacle provided. Before leaving, the hands should be washed thoroughly once again.

Immunocompromised Patients. Protective or reverse isolation is designed to protect severely immunocompromised patients, who are highly susceptible to infectious diseases that may be transmitted to them

---

TABLE 3–5 • Gowning Technique

1. Wash hands thoroughly
2. Put the gown on with the opening in the back; if a sterile gown is needed, only the inside of the gown should be touched as it is being put on.
3. Tie the strings in the back, at the neck and the waist.
4. The sleeves should be pulled down to the wrists.
5. Before removing the gown, wash hands thoroughly again.
6. To remove, untie the neck and then the waist of the gown.
7. The gown should be removed and folded with the contaminated side facing inward.
8. Place the folded gown in the specified receptacle.
9. Wash hands once more.

TABLE 3-6 • Mask and Glove Techniques

Mask technique
1. Remove a mask from the box.
2. Place the mask over the nose and mouth.
3. First tie the upper tie high on the head to keep the mask in place; then tie the lower tie.
4. The mask should be removed after removing the gown and washing the hands again thoroughly.
5. Touch only the strings when removing the mask.
6. Discard in the designated receptacle.

Glove technique
1. Gloves are put on last and removed first.
2. Gloves need not be sterile.
3. Pull the ends of the gloves over the sleeves of the gown if a gown is required.
4. Jewelry, such as rings, that might puncture a glove should be removed.
5. Gloves should be discarded after each patient.
6. Hands should be washed after the gloves are removed.
7. Gloves are worn for all contact with blood and other body fluids.

---

by other persons. Immunocompromised patients include bone marrow transplant patients, burn victims, leukemia patients, chemotherapy recipients, and organ transplant patients. Persons entering these areas or rooms should be gowned, gloved, and masked and should take with them only that equipment needed to perform the procedure. In some instances only presterilized materials may be taken into these rooms.

Intensive Care Units. These units care for the most seriously ill patients. Some patients may have an infectious disease and therefore are normally kept in a separate section of the unit, whereas other patients are recovering from surgical procedures and are being given drugs that reduce their ability to combat infection. Phlebotomists as well as other health care providers should determine the need for barrier precautions other than gloves, which should always be worn, before they approach patients.

BLOOD CULTURE COLLECTION AND BACTEREMIA

Phlebotomists play a key role in the prompt and accurate isolation of the etiologic agents in cases of **bacteremia.** Bacteremia is one of the most critical aspects of an infectious disease. The identification of the agents of bacteremia is a primary function of the clinical microbiology laboratory. The ability of the laboratory to perform this task well is directly influenced by the quality of specimens submitted. The phlebotomists who collect the blood cultures determine the quality of these critical specimens. Numerous cases of bacteremia occur each year, and the associated mortality rate may be as high as 50%. *S. aureus* and *Escherichia coli* are the two microorganisms most commonly recovered from cultures of blood. The number of bacteria circulating in the patient's blood is usually low, and the blood culture systems used are designed to amplify the number of bacteria for easier detection. False-positive results caused by contamination result in prolonged patient hospitalizations, unnecessary and expensive antibiotic treatment, and additional costs for laboratory testing. There is a lower contamination rate and greater consistency in technique in those institutions where trained phlebotomists collect the blood cultures.

Careful preparation of the patient's arm is the most critical step. The skin is normally colonized by microorganisms such as staphylococci, streptococci, corynebacteria, and bacilli. The procedure for preparation of the site (see Chapter 6) is designed to destroy the organisms present on the skin so that they are not introduced into the culture system, amplified, and reported as a positive finding. The alcohol used kills bacteria and cleans the dirt and skin debris from the pores. Povidone-iodine (Betadine) or plain iodine is applied next, and also acts to kill most of the normal skin flora. Once the site has been prepared, the phlebotomist must ensure that the site is not touched unless sterile gloves are worn.

Of all the factors that influence the successful recovery of bacteria from the blood, the most important is the volume of blood collected for each culture. Phlebotomists must be familiar with the culture system used at their institution and the recommended volume of blood to be collected. Phlebotomists play an important role in patient care, and collection of blood specimens for cultures is perhaps their most important service to their patients.

R E V I E W   Q U E S T I O N S

1. ___HANDWASHING___ is the most effective preventive measure to eliminate the transmission of disease in health care institutions.

2. Infection with ___HEPATITIS C___ is now the leading reason for liver transplantation.

3. Postexposure treatment for HIV exposure includes ZDV, 3TC, and a ___PROTEASE INHIBITOR___.

4. The use of NIOSH-approved ___RESPIRATORS___ is required for health professionals where there is a high risk of exposure to TB.

5. Most accidental needlestick injuries occur while attempting to ___RECAP___ a used needle.

6. Careful preparation of the venipuncture site is critical to reducing contamination with the ___MICROORGANISMS___ that normally colonize the skin.

References

1. Lanphear, B. (1994). Trends and patterns in the transmission of bloodborne pathogens to health care workers. *Epidemiologic Reviews,* 16(2), 437–449.
2. Centers for Disease Control. (1991). Update on adult immunization—recommendation of the Immunization Practices Advisory Committee (ACIP). *MMWR,* 40(RR-12), 5–7.
3. Gerberding, J. (1994). Incidence and prevalence of human immunodeficiency virus, hepatitis B virus, hepatitis C virus, and cytomegalovirus among health care personnel at risk for blood exposure: Final report from a longitudinal study. *The Journal of Infectious Diseases,* 170:1410–1417.
4. Centers for Disease Control and Prevention. (1997). Recommendations for follow-up of health-care workers after occupational exposure to hepatitis C virus. *MMWR,* 46(26), 603–606.

5. Centers for Disease Control and Prevention. (1996). Update: Provisional public health service recommendations for chemoprophylaxis after occupational exposure to HIV. *MMWR*, 45(22), 468–472.
6. Centers for Disease Control and Prevention. (1994). Guidelines for preventing the transmission of tuberculosis in health-care facilities. *MMWR*, 43(RR-13), 1–132.
7. Department of Health and Human Services, Department of Labor. (1995). Respiratory protective devices: Final rules and notice. *Federal Register*, 60(110), 30336–30402.
8. Hospital Infection Control Practices Advisory Committee. (1995). Recommendations for preventing the spread of vancomycin resistance. *MMWR*, 44 (RR-12), 1–13.

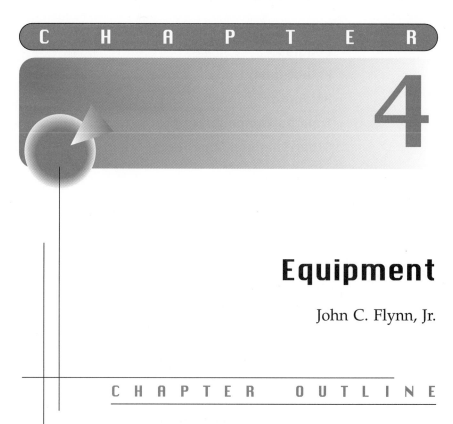

Equipment

John C. Flynn, Jr.

CHAPTER OUTLINE

- Gloves
- Goggles
- Phlebotomy Trays
- Phlebotomy Chairs
- Training Equipment
- Other Common Supplies

Phlebotomists often hear that a blood test result can only be as good as the collected specimen. This includes, in addition to proper collection technique, proper evacuated tube and needle selection. If a hematology specimen is collected in a chemistry tube, then the sample is going to be worthless for hematologic analysis. Therefore, it is very important that the correct tube, along with the proper additive, is used in every blood collection.

This chapter will discuss the various tubes, their anticoagulants, and the other common equipment associated with phlebotomy and micro-collection procedures. Before proceeding, however, the phlebotomist must understand the difference between plasma, serum, and whole blood. Plasma and serum are the liquid portion of a centrifuged blood sample. Plasma, which is collected in anticoagulated tubes, contains all coagulation factors. Serum remains after blood has clotted. It lacks some coagulation factors that were used during the clotting process. Whole blood is anticoagulated blood that has not been separated into plasma and cells via centrifugation. For example, blood collected into lavender-top tubes and used for CBC is whole blood.

TUBES AND ANTICOAGULANTS

LAVENDER-STOPPERED TUBES

In the hematology laboratory, the majority of specimens are collected in *lavender-stoppered* (or purple-stoppered) tubes. The primary additive in these tubes is the anticoagulant ethylenediaminetetra-acetate (**EDTA**). EDTA prevents blood from clotting by chelating or binding calcium. Calcium is needed for clot formation, and by binding calcium, coagulation can be prevented.

Lavender-stoppered tubes are used for general hematologic studies such as the complete blood cell **(CBC)** count, white blood cell **(WBC) differential,** and platelet count and function tests. Ideally, the blood smear for the WBC differential should be made from a drop of blood collected via a finger stick. However, this is usually not practical, and the EDTA tube is used. The smear should be made within ½ hour of the collection, because EDTA may cause some distortion of WBC morphology.

BLUE-STOPPERED TUBES

Another common tube used for the hematology laboratory (or, more precisely, the coagulation laboratory) is the *blue-stoppered* tube. Sodium citrate is used as the primary ingredient in these tubes to prevent coagulation. Sodium citrate, like EDTA, binds calcium and thus prevents coagulation. Blue-stoppered tubes are used for coagulation studies such as **prothrombin time** (PT) and **activated partial thromboplastin time** (PTT). Blood from these tubes cannot be used for CBC counts or differentials because of the effects of citrate on the cellular components.

GREEN-STOPPERED TUBES

Green-stoppered tubes contain the anticoagulant sodium heparin or lithium heparin. Heparin is a natural anticoagulant and stops the coagulation process by inactivating thrombin and thromboplastin. Blood collected in these tubes is assayed when plasma or whole blood is needed—as, for example, in tests for ammonia. Green-stoppered tubes are also the tube of choice when doing human leukocyte antigen (HLA) typing or chromosome analysis.

GRAY-STOPPERED TUBES

To inhibit glycolytic action, sodium fluoride or sodium fluoride with thymol may be used. One of these ingredients is often combined with potassium oxalate, which inhibits the clotting process by binding calcium. These ingredients are found in *gray-stoppered* evacuation tubes. Blood collected in these tubes is generally used for glucose analysis or when whole blood is needed.

YELLOW-STOPPERED TUBES

Yellow-stoppered tubes often contain acid-citrate-dextrose (ACD). In addition to inhibiting the coagulation process, ACD maintains red blood cell viability. Yellow-stoppered tubes may also contain sodium poly-anetholesulfonate (SPS). Tubes with SPS are often the tube of choice for blood culture collections.

RED-STOPPERED TUBES AND "TIGER TOPS"

Tubes with *red-stoppers* are used very frequently. These tubes have no additive and are used when serum is required for testing, such as in blood banking procedures and many serology procedures. A special type of red-stoppered tube contains a serum-cell separator. These tubes have stoppers that are red and green, and they are often referred to as "tiger tops," "speckled reds," or "mottled tops." The separator, which is a gel, works by settling between the clot and the serum during centrifugation, thereby making it easier for the laboratory worker to access the serum. The gel separates the two components of the specimen because its density is between that of the clot and serum's. See Figure 4–1. The tubes are used frequently in chemistry for a wide variety of tests. Becton-Dickinson (Rutherford, NJ) has marketed a tube with a serum-cell gel separator and a dry clot enhancer coated on the inside of the tube. Although the stopper is red, it has a gold plastic cap over it; otherwise it is used like the more traditional "tiger top" tube. This cap is referred to as a Hemoguard and will be discussed further at the end of this section.

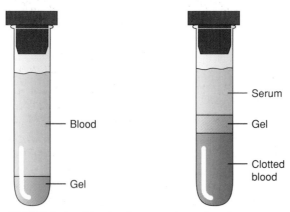

FIGURE 4-1 • Blood collection tube with gel separator.

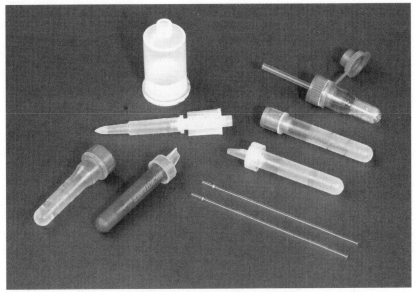

FIGURE 4-2 • Microcollection tubes.

TUBES WITH OTHER COLORED STOPPERS

Occasionally, tubes with other colored stoppers, such as black and dark blue, may be used. These may come with a variety of additives, so the phlebotomist should be aware of the additive these tubes contain before using them to collect a blood specimen. See the color plate for a listing of common stopper colors, anticoagulants, mode of action, and tests ordered.

TUBE SIZE

Tubes may come in a variety of sizes, from 15 ml down to capillary sizes for microcapillary collections. The actual volume of blood collected is dependent on the vacuum. For many tests that use a tube with an anticoagulant, a minimum amount of blood must be drawn into the tube. Otherwise the blood-to-anticoagulant ratio will not be ideal and this could adversely affect the test. The phlebotomist should check the manufacturer's specifications regarding the minimal acceptable amount of blood that can be drawn into an anticoagulated tube.

Most tubes used for adults will range from 3 to 10 ml. Pediatric evacuated tubes generally range from 2 to 4 ml. Blood-holding devices for microcapillary collection hold less than 1 ml of blood. Figure 4–2 shows some examples of blood-collecting devices for microcapillary collection. Please note, microcapillary collection is not dependent on vacuum, rather capillary action.

SPLASHGUARDS

In an effort to reduce the aerosol mist that may be generated when a stopper is removed from a tube, a stopper has been manufactured that has a plastic splashguard placed over the rubber stopper. A tube with this type of stopper is known as a Hemoguard (Fig. 4–3). Hemoguard tubes are available as replacements for all of the commonly used traditional tubes. The splashguard decreases the aerosol mist, which may be infectious. Also, some tubes are designed so that certain instruments can access the specimen directly, thus entirely eliminating the need to remove the stopper.

NEEDLES

A very important part of the blood collection system is the needle. Needles are hollow stainless steel shafts with a beveled end. Each needle is sterilized and individually packaged. In many countries needles are reused after cleaning and sterilization, but in the United States all needles are used once and then disposed of properly.

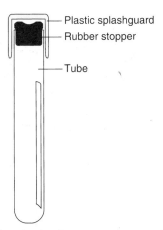

— Plastic splashguard
— Rubber stopper

— Tube

FIGURE 4-3 • Cross section of a collection tube with a splashguard, which is used to reduce the potentially infectious aerosol mist that may be generated when the stopper is removed from the tube.

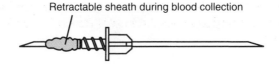

Retractable sheath during blood collection

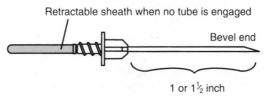

Retractable sheath when no tube is engaged

Bevel end

1 or 1½ inch

FIGURE 4-4 • Multidraw needle demonstrating the retractable sheath.

NEEDLE SIZE

Needles come in a variety of sizes, which is referred to as the *needle gauge*. The gauge is a measurement of the diameter of the needle: the larger the gauge number, the smaller the diameter of the needle. For routine phlebotomy, most needles are 21 or 22 gauge; however, during blood donation, an 18-gauge needle is common. If a patient has small or fragile veins, the phlebotomist will want to use a small gauge (for example, a 22-gauge needle).

Needles are generally 1 or 1½ inches in length. The needle selected will depend on the individual patient and on the depth of the vein from which blood is to be collected.

MULTIPLE-DRAW NEEDLES

Another variable in needle choice is whether the needle will be used for a single draw or multiple draw. In other words, will one or more than one tube of blood be collected? The multiple-draw needle has a retractable sheath over the part of the needle that extends into the evacuated tube. This sheath prevents blood from leaking out while the phlebotomist is changing tubes. Figure 4–4 demonstrates how a multiple-draw needle works.

BUTTERFLY NEEDLES

Although generally used as part of an intravenous set to administer fluids or medicine to patients, the butterfly needle (Fig. 4–5) is sometimes used to collect blood from difficult patients. Once the butterfly needle is

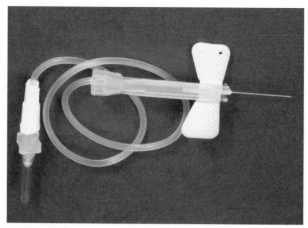

FIGURE 4-5 • Winged infusion set, commonly referred to as a butterfly.

in place, a syringe or evacuated tube, with a tube holder, is used to withdraw blood from the vein. See Chapter 5.

BLOOD LANCETS

For difficult patients, including situations that normally call for microcapillary techniques, a blood lancet may be used. This is a small, sterile, disposable instrument used for skin puncture (Fig. 4–6). Lancets are available with a variety of point lengths to help control the depth of puncture, which is especially important in children and infants. A variety of semiautomated lancet devices are commercially available, but the manual lancet is the most commonly used device for microcapillary puncture.

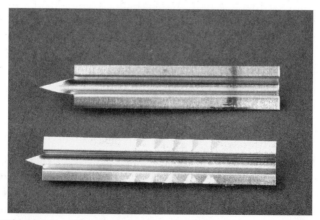

FIGURE 4-6 • Microlances; notice the difference in point lengths.

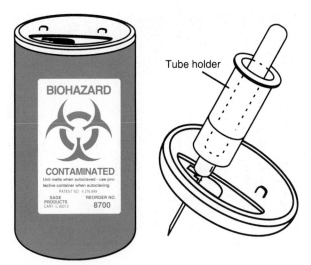

FIGURE 4-7 • Needle disposal container. The inset shows the hub of the needle seated into the lid. The needle is unscrewed and allowed to drop into the receptacle, which can be permanently closed when filled.

NEEDLE DISPOSAL EQUIPMENT

Needle disposal equipment has evolved over time from manually recapping and then unscrewing needles, to cutting off the needle, to unscrewing the needle directly into a puncture-proof container and even to the point of discarding both the needle and tube holder. The purpose is to avoid any accidental needle punctures, and therefore, the less the phlebotomist has to directly manipulate the needle, the less possibility there is of needle puncture. The puncture-proof containers come in a variety of sizes; some are small enough to fit conveniently on the phlebotomist's tray. Figure 4–7 demonstrates how the needle is unscrewed into a disposal container. Other needle safety and disposal devices are commercially available to prevent accidental needle punctures. See Figure 4–8.

TUBE HOLDERS

The tube holder, or, as it is sometimes called, the barrel or adapter, allows the phlebotomist to safely and securely manipulate the evacuated tubes and draw blood from a patient. Holders come in a variety of sizes to accomodate normal and pediatric size evacuated tubes. See Figure 4–9. Figure 4–10 shows a fully assembled needle, tube, and tube holder.

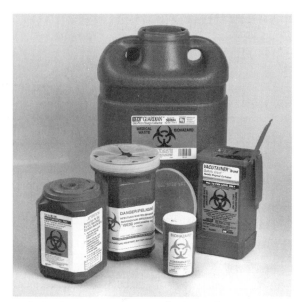

FIGURE 4-8 • Various needle disposal containers.

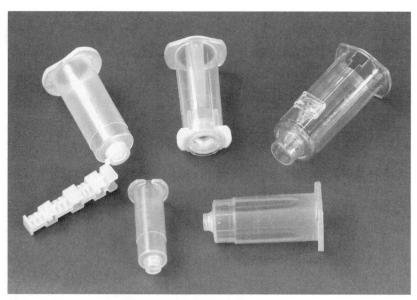

FIGURE 4-9 • Various tube holders.

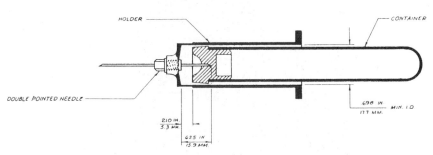

POSITION 1
PREPARATION FOR VENIPUNCTURE

HOLDER

CONTAINER

DOUBLE POINTED NEEDLE

.698 IN
17.7 MM.   MIN. I.D.

.210 IN.
5.3 MM.

.625 IN
15.9 MM.

NOTES:

1 NEEDLE TO LOCK IN PLACE WITH MATING HOLDER

2 STOPPER DIMENSIONS TO ALLOW FOR TWO
   POSITIONS AS SHOWN.

POSITION 2
COLLECTION OF SPECIMEN

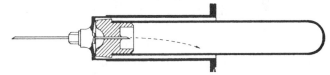

FIGURE 4-10A • Line drawing of assembled venipuncture set. (Reproduced with permission from H1-A4, "Evacuated Tubes and Additives for Blood Specimen Collection—Fourth Edition; Approved Standard," NCCLS, 940 West Valley Road, Suite 1400, Wayne, PA 19087, U.S.A., 1996.)

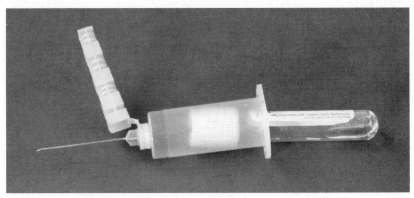

FIGURE 4-10B • Fully assembled venipuncture set.

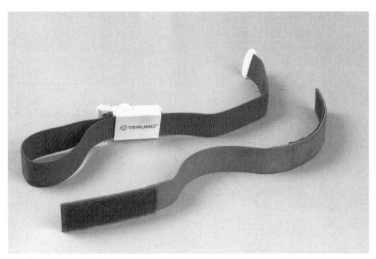

FIGURE 4-11 • In addition to the traditional latex tourniquet, the illustration shows two other varieties.

TOURNIQUETS

The purpose of the tourniquet is to increase resistance in the venous blood flow. When this happens, the veins become distended and can be more easily palpated or located. However, the tourniquet should not remain on the patient too long (1 to 2 minutes maximum), resulting in hemoconcentration (see Chapter 7), because this could adversely affect the test results as well as be uncomfortable and/or harm the patient. There are a variety of tourniquets available, including blood pressure cuffs, rubber tubing, and rubber straps.

Although a blood pressure cuff is an ideal tourniquet because the pressure can be accurately regulated, it is not practical to use for routine venipunctures. However, when confronted with a difficult "stick," a blood pressure cuff is very helpful. The more commonly used tourniquet is the rubber strap, which is tied in a slip loop (see Chapter 5) above the venipuncture site. Some rubber straps are equipped with Velcro, thereby eliminating the need for the slip loop. Penrose tubing is occasionally used, but the rubber strap is generally the tourniquet of choice. See Figure 4–11 for two types of tourniquets.

GLOVES

With the implementation of the Occupational Safety and Health Administration (OSHA) regulations for blood-borne pathogens and the advent of Universal Precautions now incorporated in Standard Precautions, gloves have become mandatory in blood collection. They provide a protective barrier between the phlebotomist and any infectious agents that could enter the body through a cut or abrasion. Remember, just because cuts or abrasions cannot be seen does not mean they are not present. *There is no excuse for not using gloves.*

Gloves are made from a variety of materials, but the most commonly used materials are vinyl, latex, and nitrile. Vinyl gloves are probably the least desirable, because they do not fit snugly and do not conform to the shape of the individual's hand. Latex gloves are the most commonly used, because they fit nicely and conform to the individual's hand. Many phlebotomists prefer the nitrile gloves. These have a fit similar to that of latex gloves but are more tear resistant and feel more comfortable on the hand. However, they are slightly more expensive.

Commonly, gloves are available with talcum powder lightly dusted inside them, which makes it easier for the wearer to put them on and take them off. However, some individuals develop allergies to the powder, and occasionally the powder may interfere with some tests or be harmful to sensitive equipment. For these situations, powder-free gloves are available from a variety of vendors. Others are allergic to latex and must use non-latex gloves or a glove liner.

Finally, gloves are available in dispenser boxes or are individually wrapped and sterilized, which is more costly. Generally, dispenser boxes are most commonly encountered in phlebotomy units.

GOGGLES

Safety goggles are now recommended for use during phlebotomy procedures. They are to prevent splashing or aerosol from possibly exposing the phlebotomist's eyes to bloodborne pathogens. Regular glasses are not acceptable substitutes for safety goggles.

PHLEBOTOMY TRAYS

Phlebotomy trays are commercially available carriers that enable phlebotomists to conveniently carry all the equipment and supplies they may need to perform their job. These trays are generally carried, but some hospitals provide phlebotomists with push carts on which they may place their trays. The trays must allow the phlebotomist to carry an adequate supply of all of the previously mentioned equip-

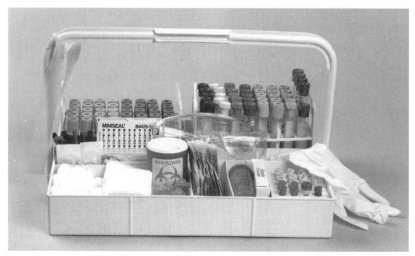

FIGURE 4-12 • Fully stocked phlebotomy tray.

ment. See Figure 4–12 for a picture of a fully stocked phlebotomy tray.

PHLEBOTOMY CHAIRS

A final piece of equipment worth mentioning is the phlebotomy chair. These are most often found in outpatient blood-collecting areas. There are several models available from manufacturers. However, they all provide a sturdy backrest, support for the arm, and a restraint system to keep the patient from falling out. They also generally have storage areas for tubes, needles, etc. Figure 4–13 shows an acceptable phlebotomy chair. Some phlebotomy chairs recline so that patients may lie down if they feel weak.

TRAINING EQUIPMENT

All the equipment mentioned so far is used in both the actual practice of phlebotomy as well as teaching phlebotomy students. However, there is equipment that is used specifically for training in most phlebotomy training programs. At one time, venipuncture training may have consisted of having students stick oranges or chicken legs; now, simulated arms and hands—complete with "blood"—are available from various manufacturers (Fig. 4–14). Manikins are also available for teaching students how to hold infants for microcapillary collection.

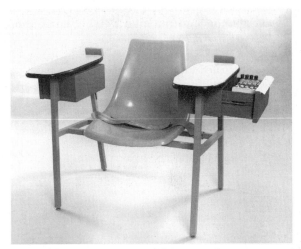

FIGURE 4-13 • Phlebotomy chair.

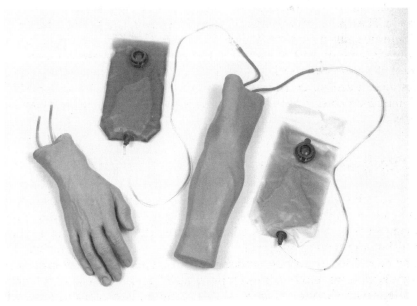

FIGURE 4-14 • Phlebotomy training aids.

TABLE 4-1 • Common Equipment a Phlebotomist Should Carry

Needles (various sizes and microcapillary)
Evacuated tubes (various sizes and colors)
Microcapillary collection equipment
Tube holders
Tourniquets
Alcohol swabs
Gauze
Adhesive bandages or tape
Gloves
Sharps containers
Marking pens
Clay sealer
Goggles

OTHER COMMON SUPPLIES

Other common supplies that the phlebotomist will need are alcohol pads, gauze, surgical tape, pens, ammonia salts, and adhesive bandages. Table 4–1 lists the common equipment that a phlebotomist may need.

REVIEW QUESTIONS

1. The anticoagulant in a lavender top tube is (EDTA).
   Ethelene diaminotetraacetic acid.

2. A small, sterile, disposable instrument used for skin puncture is the _LANCET_ (autolet).

3. _NEEDLES_
   are disposed of in puncture-proof containers.

4. The rubber strap is a type of _TOURNIQUET_.

5. In an effort to reduce aerosol mist, a _____
   SPLASH GUARD
   is placed over the rubber stopper by some manufacturers.

6. Cells and serum are separated on the basis of _DENSITY_ in tubes with gel separators.

7. _GOGGLES_
   prevent aerosol from possibly exposing blood-borne pathogens to the phlebotomist via the eyes.

5

Proper Procedures for Venipuncture

John C. Flynn, Jr.

The previous chapter discussed the equipment and anticoagulants used in common blood collection techniques. In this chapter, the actual techniques practiced in evacuated tube and microcapillary collections, beginning with greeting and identifying the patient and continuing through to labeling and transporting the specimen, will be discussed and illustrated. (Syringe collection technique will be discussed in a subsequent chapter.)

PATIENT GREETING AND IDENTIFICATION

The manner in which a phlebotomist greets a patient can often set the tone for the remainder of the phlebotomy procedure. A later chapter is devoted to interpersonal communication and professionalism, but it must be emphasized here that phlebotomists must always conduct themselves in a professional manner. Therefore, when greeting a patient, be courteous and respectful. Treat them the way you would like to be treated. Additionally, if the patient's door is shut when you get to the room, knock and listen for a response before you enter. Of course, this may not always be feasible, depending on the patient and the surrounding circumstances.

When greeting the patient, the phlebotomist must identify him- or herself and tell the patient why he or she is there. One of the most important steps in venipuncture—possibly the most important—is proper patient identification. Identification can be both visual and verbal. When you enter a patient's room, in addition to the test requisition, you will generally have certain information such as the patient's name, identification number, and age or date of birth. Compare the information you have with the patient's physical appearance and the identification bracelet. For example, if your requisition lists the patient's name as Sarah Jones and you encounter a male patient, there is a problem. Furthermore, do not use the information on the chart that is attached to the bed or on the name plate on or above the bed. Patients may be transferred, and name plates may not be accurate. The only dependable information is on the patient's wristband. Also, it is best to ask patients to state their name rather than having them respond to a question. For example, it is best to say, "Please tell me your full name," rather than, "Are you Mrs. Jones?" If the patient is incoherent or has difficulty hearing, they may answer "yes," no matter what they are asked, in an effort to be cooperative.

ROUTINE VENIPUNCTURE

This section will discuss the proper procedure for performing routine venipuncture. Remember, as in the illustrations, *gloves must be worn at all times.* Also, see the Venipuncture Competency Evaluation at the end of this chapter following the Review Questions.

POSITIONING AND TOURNIQUET APPLICATION (Fig. 5–1).

Position the patient's arm in such a way that it is comfortable for both you and the patient, allowing clear access to the antecubital area. The arm should be supported by a firm surface such as an armrest on a phlebotomy chair or on the bed if the patient is lying down. It is courteous to ask the patient if he or she has an arm preference for the venipuncture, but the ultimate decision rests with the phlebotomist. Once the arm is positioned, place the tourniquet firmly about the upper arm. The tourniquet needs to be tight enough to increase blood pressure in the veins but not so tight that it cuts off the circulation. Figure 5–2 shows how the tourniquet should be tied. After some practice, you will learn how to adjust the tourniquet for proper snugness. The tourniquet should never remain on the patient's arm for more than 1 to 2 minutes.

CHOOSING THE SITE (Fig. 5–3).

Try to locate the median cubital vein (generally the largest and best anchored vein, near the center of the antecubital area). Other veins that may be acceptable are the cephalic and the basilic veins

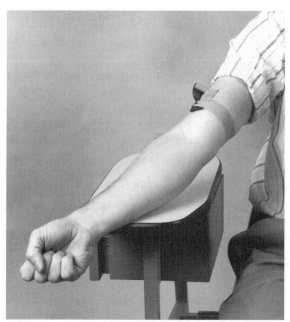

FIGURE 5-1 • A properly supported arm with tourniquet.

Proper method for tying a tourniquet

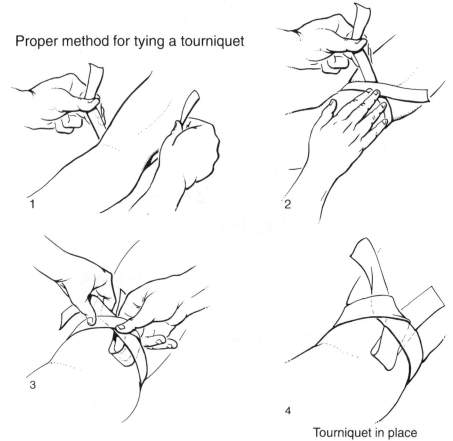

1

2

3

4

Tourniquet in place

FIGURE 5-2 • Tourniquet application.

(see Figure 5–3B). Veins in the back of the hand may also be acceptable, but in these cases it is wise to use pediatric needles and evacuated tubes or a "butterfly." (This will be discussed later.) To enhance visualization of the veins, position the arm at a downward angle, using the force of gravity as an aid. Also, rubbing the forearm toward the antecubital area and instructing the patient to make a fist may enhance vein visualization. Palpating and feeling for the vein with the forefinger is also helpful; do not forget that you can look on both arms before a decision is made and that there will be times when you cannot see the vein but can feel it. The prospective venipuncture site should be free of skin abrasions, lesions, and scar tissue.

ASSEMBLING THE EQUIPMENT

3

Assemble the needle, the barrel, and the first tube you wish to use as in Figures 4–9 and 5–4. The needle should not be uncovered until ready to perform venipuncture. Place any additional tubes to be used in a convenient location, keeping some spares handy. The gauze, alcohol pads, and bandages should be ready. (*Note:* Some phlebotomists may elect to do this step before applying the tourniquet; this is preferable.)

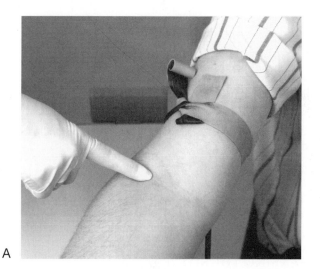

A

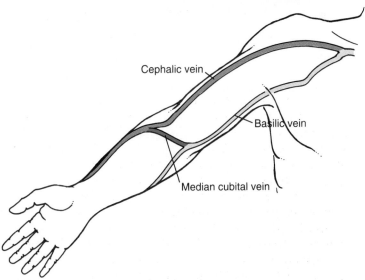

Cephalic vein

Basilic vein

Median cubital vein

B

FIGURE 5-3 • *A* and *B*. Locating a vein.

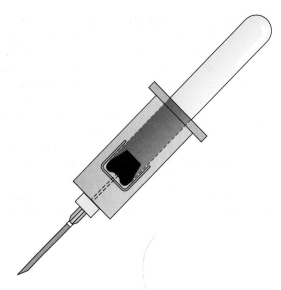

FIGURE 5-4 • An assembled needle, holder, and tube; note that needle is uncovered.

CLEANSING THE SITE (Fig. 5–5).

Cleanse the venipuncture site with 70% isopropyl alcohol by making outward concentric circles. *This must be allowed to dry, either by air drying or by using clean gauze. Failure to do so could result in red cell hemolysis in the collected sample and discomfort to the patient. Once the site is cleansed, it must not be touched;* if touched, it must be recleansed.

PERFORMING THE VENIPUNCTURE (Fig. 5–6).

With the bevel up, quickly and smoothly insert the needle into the vein at approximately a 15° angle and engage the evacuated tube.

*(**Special Note:** There is no right way or wrong way to hold the needle and adapter for venipuncture. Phlebotomy instructors may advocate one way over another because of familiarity and experience. The phlebotomy student must discover which way is most comfortable and which yields the best results.)*

Be sure to stretch the skin surrounding the venipuncture site before inserting the needle; this will aid in anchoring the vein and will make needle insertion less painful. Anchor the vein by gently stretching the skin below the venipuncture site. Do not "straddle" the site with a thumb and finger; this increases the chance of inadvertently sticking yourself. Never tell patients that they will not feel the needle puncture or that it will not hurt. Be honest with the patient. If no blood is immediately forthcoming, slight manipulation of the needle may be helpful; you may have gone in too deep, not deep enough, or to one side of the vein. Avoid "probing," and do not attempt a venipuncture more than two times on a given patient. (See Chapter 7 for a more thorough discussion on what to do if you do not obtain blood.)

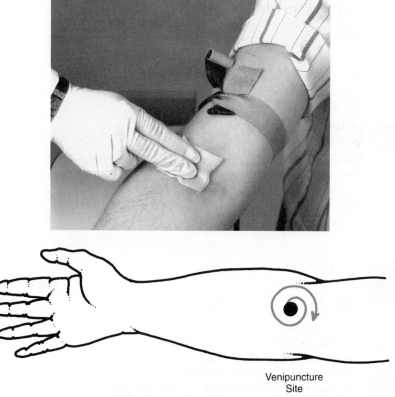

Venipuncture
Site

FIGURE 5-5 • Cleansing the venipuncture site from the center out.

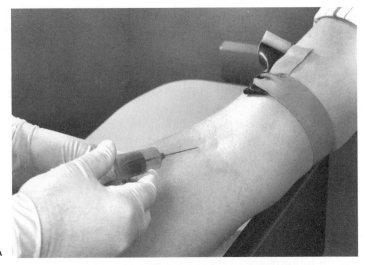

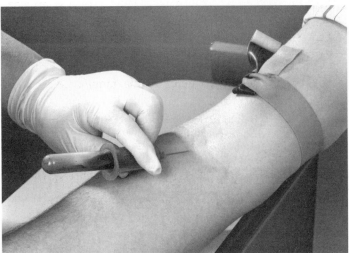

FIGURE 5-6 • *A* and *B.* Venipuncture.

6

RELEASING THE TOURNIQUET (Fig. 5–7).

Once good blood flow is established and before the final tube is filled, release the tourniquet. If the tourniquet was applied properly, you should be able to release it with a simple tug.

7

REMOVING THE NEEDLE (Fig. 5–8).

Once the last tube of blood is filled and you have removed it from the needle and tube holder, you may remove the needle. Do this in a single smooth, swift motion, and quickly apply clean gauze over the puncture site. If the patient is able, instruct him or her to apply pressure and to keep the arm straight. If the patient is unable to do this, it is the phlebotomist's responsibility to apply pressure until the bleeding has stopped. Outpatients may use a bandage to cover the venipuncture site, but hospitals may have different policies about using bandages on inpatients. Be sure you are familiar with the policies at your institution.

8 **NEEDLE DISPOSAL** (Fig. 5–9).
Properly dispose of your needle in an approved disposal unit. *Do not lay it down, and do not recap it.*

9 **SPECIMEN LABELING AND TRANSPORTATION** (Fig. 5–10).
Immediately label the specimen. If any specimens require mixing (e.g., in blue- or purple-stoppered tubes or any anticoagulated tube), do so by gently inverting the tubes several times. Regarding labeling, remember that the patient's wristband is the primary source of information. In some hospitals, certain specimens (e.g., those for the blood bank) must be hand labeled and initialed by the phlebotomist. Therefore, be familiar with any special labeling requirements at your institution. Also, as a responsible phlebotomist, you must be aware of any special transportation

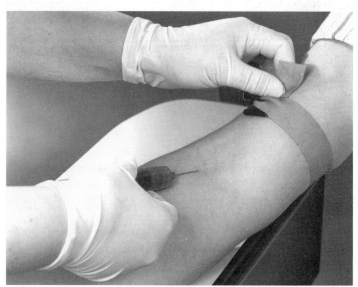

FIGURE 5-7 • Releasing the tourniquet when the last tube of blood is nearly full.

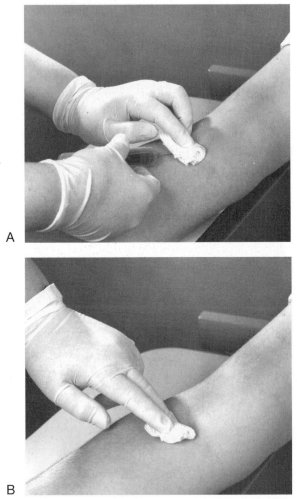

A

B

FIGURE 5-8 • *A,* Removing the needle with gauze lightly applied over site. *B,* Apply pressure after needle removal.

requirements. Does the specimen need to be transported on ice (e.g., for an ammonia test)? Does the specimen need to be maintained at 37°C (e.g., for a cold agglutinin test)? Is the specimen a STAT (i.e., needing immediate analysis)? Be familiar with any special transportation requirements before collecting the blood specimen.

10 HAND WASHING
Before moving on to the next patient, remove and properly discard your gloves, and then thoroughly wash your hands as was discussed in Chapter 3.

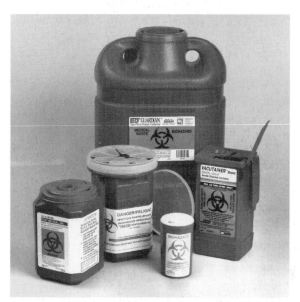

FIGURE 5-9 • Needle disposal units.

Occasionally, venipuncture must be performed on a young child or toddler. The equipment and procedure are basically the same as for an adult patient, but the child may need some restraint. See Chapter 7 for further discussion and illustration of performing phlebotomy on a child.

MICROCAPILLARY BLOOD COLLECTION

Microcapillary blood collections are used primarily when the patient has no adequate veins for venipuncture, either because of age (very young or very old) or for some other reason, such as burns or dermatitis. Obviously the amount of blood collected will be much smaller than that collected via venipuncture, which in turn means the physician must be very sure of the tests he or she wishes to be performed.

FIGURE 5-10 • Properly labeled specimen which includes: patient name, ID number, date and time specimen collected, and phlebotomist ID (in this case initials).

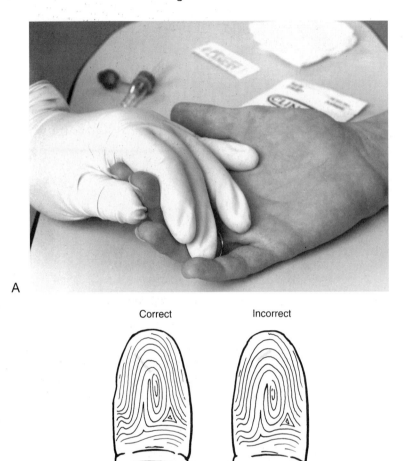

Correct   Incorrect

B

FIGURE 5-11 • *A,* An accepted way to hold a finger for skin puncture. *B,* The skin puncture in a finger stick should be perpendicular to the lines of the fingerprint.

The technique for microcapillary collection is not drastically different from the venipuncture technique described earlier. Gloves are used at all times. The site of the skin puncture is usually the finger but may also be the earlobe or the heel in the case of an infant (discussed further in Chapter 6). No tourniquet is applied, but instead the site is held firmly by the phlebotomist. Figure 5–11*A* shows how to hold a finger to perform a skin puncture. Site preparation (Fig. 5–12) is identical, but a microlance is used instead of a needle and tube (see Fig. 5–13). When doing a finger stick, make the puncture off the center of the finger and perpendicular to the lines of the fingerprint (Fig. 5–11*B*). It is important to remember to

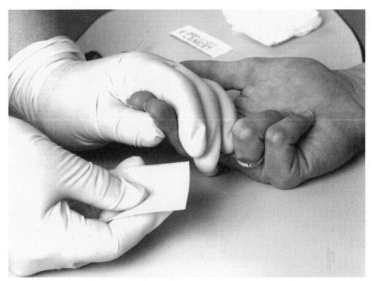

FIGURE 5-12 • Site preparation for finger stick.

wipe away the first drop of blood, because the blood in this drop will be diluted with tissue fluid, which could alter the laboratory results (See Fig. 5–14). Some variation of a microcollection tube is used to collect the blood (see Fig. 5–15). At the completion of the blood collection, either the

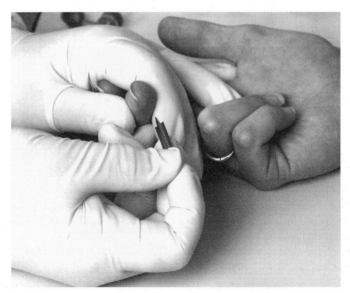

FIGURE 5-13 • Finger stick using a microlance.

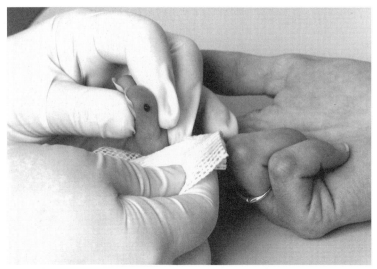

FIGURE 5-14 • Wiping away the first drop of blood.

phlebotomist or the patient must maintain pressure on the puncture site until bleeding has stopped (Fig. 5–16). All used material is properly disposed of—the lancet in the puncture-proof container and the used gauze and gloves in a biohazard receptacle. As in venipuncture, hands

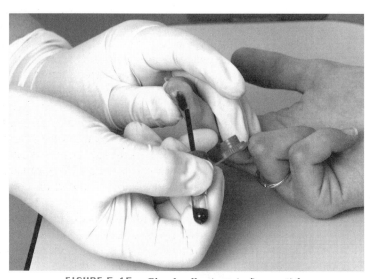

FIGURE 5-15 • Blood collection via finger stick.

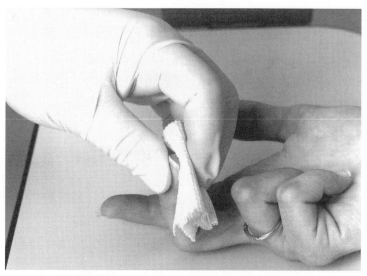

FIGURE 5-16 • Applying pressure after collection.

must be washed before going to the next patient. See the Capillary Blood Collection Competency Evaluation at the end of this chapter following the Review Questions.

VENIPUNCTURE USING A BUTTERFLY SET

A butterfly needle or winged infusion set may be used to access difficult veins (see Fig. 4–5). Butterflies are commonly used for pediatric or elderly patients, and a common site is the back of the hand. Butterfly needles can be used with either evacuated tube systems or with syringes. The evacuated tube system is more commonly used, especially with beginning phlebotomists.

The procedure is very similar to routine phlebotomy, including patient identification, site preparation, needle disposal, and precautions. A tourniquet is used which is usually placed around the wrist if veins on the back of the hand are going to be used. The infusion needle is carefully "threaded" into the vein. A Luer adapter on the end of the infusion set can be threaded into the tube adapter and then evacuated tubes can be filled. It is probably best to use pediatric tubes since full-size tubes may create too great a pull on the vein, leading to collapse. Extra precautions must be used when the needle is removed, since it tends to dangle and can easily cause an accident. It should be disposed of properly as soon as possible. See Figures 5–17 through 5–21 for a photographic series demonstrating the use of winged infusion sets.

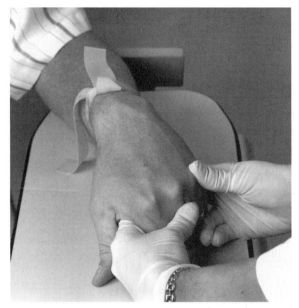

FIGURE 5-17 • Locating a vein, note the location of the tourniquet.

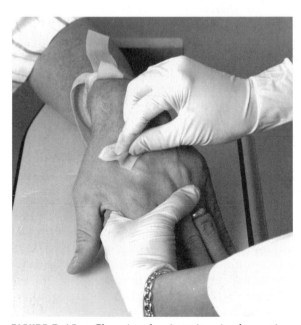

FIGURE 5-18 • Cleansing the site using circular motion.

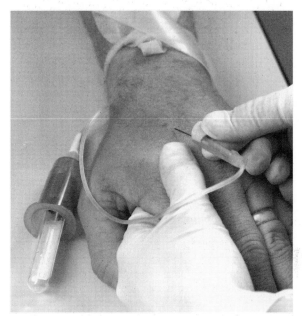

FIGURE 5-19 • Perform the puncture; note the thumb stretching the skin and anchoring the site.

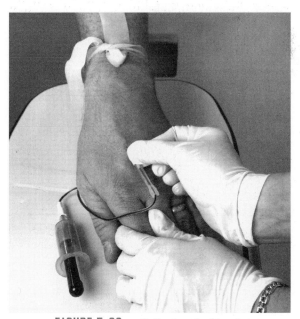

FIGURE 5-20 • Collecting the blood.

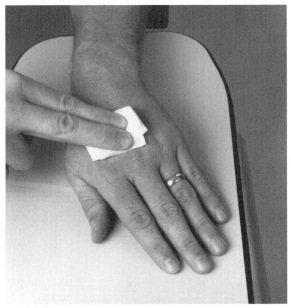

FIGURE 5-21 • Applying pressure after collection.

General Considerations

The following general considerations apply to blood collection either by venipuncture or by skin puncture.

1. Always act professionally and be considerate of the patient.
2. Never quarrel with a patient.
3. Use expendable equipment, such as needles, lancets, and gauze, only once.
4. Avoid venipuncture more than two times on a given patient.
5. Always wear gloves.
6. Never recap needles, but dispose of them properly.

ORDER OF DRAW

The order in which a phlebotomist fills tubes collected via evacuated systems is critical to ascertaining good test results. Tissue fluids may interfere with coagulation studies and skin surface bacteria may lead to false positives in blood cultures, to name a few. Additionally, additives from the tubes themselves may cause erroneous results if there should happen to be any carryover between collection tubes. For example, oxalate found in gray-topped tubes can interfere with red blood cell morphology. Therefore, the order of draw in blood collection must be done in a way to minimize these potentially interfering factors.

The commonly accepted order of draw is as follows:

1. Blood culture tubes first, generally yellow tops (if not special blood collection bottles); this minimizes the chance of bacterial contamination
2. Empty tubes, generally plain red-top tubes or with gel separators without clot enhancers
3. Additive tubes:
   a. Light blue
   b. Heparin
   c. Lavender
   d. Gray

Remember, always follow manufacturer's directions when appropriate. Furthermore, local protocol may differ regarding the order of draw especially with additive tubes, so be sure to follow your employer's standard operating procedure. Finally, if a coagulation tube (light blue) is the only one requested, collect a red-top tube prior to this one and discard it. This eliminates the possibility of interference by tissue fluids during coagulation studies (here again, check local protocol).

PHYSIOLOGIC AND BIOLOGIC CONSIDERATIONS

Occasionally, laboratory testing of a blood sample will result in a spurious result or be considered a "mistake" by a physician in the laboratory or nurse on the floor. Actually what has occurred is a variation from the **basal state** of the patient, which has influenced the **analyte.** In short, the basal state in the baseline condition of the patient prior to any treatment or medication. Any number of things can interfere with the basal state of a patient (e.g., diet, exercise, stress, trauma, or change in posture). The time of day can also interfere with the baseline results one would expect to obtain on testing.

Diet is probably the most obvious factor that may affect testing. This is especially true when analyses for glucose or triglycerides are performed. The importance of collecting fasting or timed specimens is discussed more fully in Chapter 6, but it is important to note the time a specimen is collected and whether it is a fasting specimen.

The level of certain enzymes, such as creatine phosphokinase (CPK), in the blood may help diagnose heart damage. However, this same enzyme is also found in all other muscle tissue. If the patient has engaged in moderate to strenuous *exercise* in the 24 hours preceding the collection of the blood specimen, an elevated level of the enzyme, not related to a heart condition, may be found. (It should be noted that if an elevated CPK level is encountered, a more specific test should be performed.) Exercise may also affect the levels of other enzymes as well as various hemostatic factors. For the phlebotomist, it may be wise to note whether a patient has engaged in exercise in the 24 hours preceding blood collection.

Stress caused by the anticipation of having a blood specimen collected may alter the levels of certain constituents in the blood. For example, white blood cells may increase if the patient is overanxious about the phlebotomy. Therefore, it is best—and easier—to collect the specimen when the patient is calm.

The *trauma* associated with an accident will adversely affect the results of some tests. If the muscles are injured in a traumatic accident, CPK will be released into the blood system and may initially give a false indication of heart trouble.

A change in posture may not only change blood pressure, it may also significantly alter the results obtained when testing for certain analytes such as proteins, lipids, iron, and enzymes. This is especially true when a patient has been in one position for a period of time and blood is collected shortly after he or she changes position.

Finally, the *time of day* that a specimen is collected will affect the results of testing. Serum cortisol, used to monitor adrenal function, is notably affected by circadian rhythm, again illustrating the importance of noting the time that a blood specimen is collected.

In addition to the physiologic variations mentioned earlier, certain biologic conditions may affect testing results. These include factors such as age, sex, race, and pregnancy. If appropriate, laboratories generally have different sets of normal values depending on what test is being performed. Table 5–1 shows how normal values for hemoglobin may vary. Often the age, sex, and race are noted on requisition slips or computer-generated labels. If not, it will be very informative to the laboratory if the phlebotomist provides this information, in addition to noting whether the patient is pregnant.

TABLE 5-1 • Hemoglobin Values According to Age and Gender	
	Normal Hemoglobin Value (gm/dl)
Newborn	17–23
2-month-old child	9–14
Adult male	14–18
Adult female	12–16

The above paragraphs mention only a few of the many blood constituents that may be affected by a variety of physiologic and biologic conditions. For phlebotomists, any information that can be provided to the laboratory to help explain spurious results and avoid a "laboratory error" will be a great service in saving both time and money, as well as possibly saving the patient from a needless venipuncture.

REVIEW QUESTIONS

1. Probably the most important aspect of phlebotomy is proper ___*identification*___ *Patient* .

2. The cleanser of choice for routine venipuncture is ___*70% Isopropyl Alcohol*___ .

3. The ___*tourniquet*___ should always be released before removing the needle from a vein.

4. You should always ___*wash hands + glove*___ before moving on to the next patient.

5. ___*Strenuous Exercise*___ may cause an elevation in blood enzymes.

6. Venipuncture needles are inserted at approximately a ___*15*___-degree angle.

7. A ___*BUTTERFLY*___ needle is often used in elderly and pediatric patients.

8. If no blood culture tube is collected, then an ___*PLAIN RED / empty*___ tube should be the first tube collected using an evacuated system.

VENIPUNCTURE COMPETENCY EVALUATION

Student's Name _____ Date _____

Evaluated by _____

Result of Evaluation _____

Conditions for Testing:

- A patient of any age
- Request for multiple blood samples
- Readily available equipment
- Training period for all previous labs
- Student has been given a copy of the exam before training period begins
- No references may be used or questions asked

Scoring:

1. Steps 3, 15, 21, 27, 28, and 30 (in boldface) are critical. Exam is stopped if student omits such a step. Retest is required after additional training to be specified by the instructor.
2. More than two checks in the "no" column requires a retest after additional training.

Criteria for Evaluation:

Competent ("C")	Student performs all steps as indicated and in the proper sequence. The numerical grade is 100.
Minimally Competent ("MC")	Student performs all critical steps as indicated. A maximum of two checks appear in the "no" column for the noncritical steps. The numerical grade is 80.
Incompetent ("I")	Instructor stops exam because a critical step is omitted; or more than two checks appear in the "no" column; or steps are out of sequence. The numerical grade is 60.

COMPETENCY SCORE SHEET EXPECTED OBSERVABLE PERFORMANCE For venipuncture, the student:	YES	NO
1. Wears gloves.		
2. Greets patient, puts patient at ease, explains the procedure.		
3. **Identifies patient: checks wristband, asks name, checks labels and request forms.**		
4. Positions patient: supports patient's arm, appears comfortable.		
5. Selects equipment to correspond with requested tests.		
6. Places needle on holder.		
7. Positions tube in holder without breaking vacuum.		
8. Places sponges and other tubes within reach.		
9. Reassures patient while positioning tourniquet; asks patient to clench fist.		
10. Selects vein by palpation with index finger.		
11. Cleanses area with alcohol sponge (student may repeat 8, 9, and 10).		
12. Removes needle cap.		
13. Positions bevel up.		
14. Fixes vein by placing thumb about 2 cm below site of entry and pulling skin downward to keep it taut.		
15. **Angles needle at approximately 15° without contamination.**		
16. Inserts needle under skin and into lumen about 1 cm below prominent part of vein.		
17. Pushes tube into holder without moving needle (order of draw).		
18. Obtains blood and allows tube to fill completely.		
19. Removes tube and replaces with another tube without moving needle (may repeat 18).		

The student:	YES	NO
20. Asks patient to relax fist.		
21. Removes tourniquet.		
22. When last tube is filled, pulls tube back to line on holder to seal needle.		
23. Covers site with gauze and removes needle slowly without changing angle.		
24. Applies pressure to gauze. Asks patient to hold gauze with pressure. Tells patient to keep arm straight.		
25. Removes tube from holder and mixes tubes.		
26. Removes needle from holder using safety device.		
27. Labels tubes.		
28. Discards waste in proper containers.		
29. Matches tubes to request slips.		
30. Checks patient's arm to be sure hemostasis has occurred. Asks patient if he or she is feeling all right. Tells patient not to exercise arm immediately.		
31. Places Band-Aid on arm if needed.		
32. Leaves patient safely.		

Comments:

CAPILLARY BLOOD COLLECTION COMPETENCY EVALUATION

Student's Name _____ Date _____

Evaluated by _____

Result of Evaluation _____

Conditions for Testing:

- A patient of any age
- Request for multiple blood samples
- Readily available equipment
- 3-hour lab exercise training period
- Student has been given a copy of the exam before training period begins
- No references may be used or questions asked

Scoring:

1. Steps 3, 15, 16, and 17 (in boldface) are critical. Exam is stopped if student omits such a step. Retest is required after additional training to be specified by the instructor.
2. More than two checks in the "no" column requires a retest after additional training.

Criteria for Evaluation:

Competent ("C")	Student performs all steps as indicated and in the proper sequence. The numerical grade is 100.
Minimally Competent ("MC")	Student performs all critical steps as indicated. A maximum of two checks appear in the "no" column for the noncritical steps. The numerical grade is 80.
Incompetent ("I")	Instructor stops exam because a critical step is omitted; or more than two checks appear in the "no" column; or steps are out of sequence. The numerical grade is 60.

COMPETENCY SCORE SHEET EXPECTED OBSERVABLE PERFORMANCE For capillary blood collection, the student:	YES	NO
1. Wears gloves.		
2. Greets patient, puts patient at ease, explains the procedure.		
3. **Properly identifies patient: checks wristband, asks name, checks labels and request forms.**		
4. Selects correct equipment and organizes all supplies before beginning.		
5. Selects proper site.		
6. Cleanses site with alcohol.		
7. Dries site with gauze.		
8. Punctures ball of finger with one swift motion.		
9. Wipes away first drop of blood.		
10. Massages finger gently.		
11. Holds capillary tube to blood source and allows to fill—does not touch tube to finger.		
12. Wipes excess blood from outside of capillary tube, seals it, or otherwise handles equipment according to previously specified instructions.		
13. Collects all capillary blood samples in duplicate when specified.		
14. Applies dry gauze to stop bleeding.		
15. **Labels samples.**		
16. **Checks patient's finger and applies Band-Aid if needed.**		
17. **Disposes of used equipment in appropriate manner.**		

Comments:

6

Special Collection Procedures

John C. Flynn, Jr.

A well-trained and experienced phlebotomist is a valuable asset to the clinical laboratory or any health care setting when venipuncture is performed. Often the phlebotomist is asked or required to do more than perform routine venipunctures or microcapillary collections. This chapter outlines other blood collection procedures or tests that phlebotomists may perform depending on the institution where they are employed.

BLEEDING TIME TEST

A bleeding time test is a rather simple test that is used to ascertain the functioning of a patient's platelets. Platelets are crucial in stopping capillary bleeding, and the bleeding time gives the clinician information about the integrity of the patient's platelet function. A prolonged bleeding time indicates that either the platelet count is low or the platelets are not functioning properly.

Although it is not the responsibility of phlebotomists to monitor the medications a patient may be taking, they should be aware that certain drugs will prolong the bleeding time. The most noteworthy among these drugs are aspirin and aspirin-containing compounds. Aspirin impairs platelets' ability to form aggregates. Antihistamines also interfere with bleeding time.

The Ivy method is the most popular procedure to determine bleeding time. This involves applying a sphygmomanometer (blood pressure) cuff to the upper arm and inflating it to 40 mm Hg (Fig. 6–1A). After the volar area of the arm is cleansed with 70% isopropyl alcohol, (Fig. 6-1B) small incisions are made with a commercially available, standardized instrument (Fig. 6–1C,D). Some produce two incisions while others create a single incision. Then every 30 seconds the blood is blotted, not wiped, with filter paper until bleeding is stopped (Fig. 6–1E), at which time the sphygmomanometer cuff can be released. If an instrument that causes two incisions is used, the difference between the two sites should not be more than 30 seconds. If bleeding occurs for more than 15 minutes, the cuff is released, and the results are noted simply as greater than 15 minutes. The phlebotomist should remain with the patient until bleeding stops (Fig. 6–1F). The results are recorded and returned to the laboratory.

NEONATAL BLOOD COLLECTION

With the increasing sophistication of medical testing and care, premature infants have a better chance of survival today than they did as recently as 1980. Infants as small as 2 lb or less in weight and more than 10 weeks premature are surviving. To monitor the progress of care and treatment, blood must be collected for analysis. Common neonatal

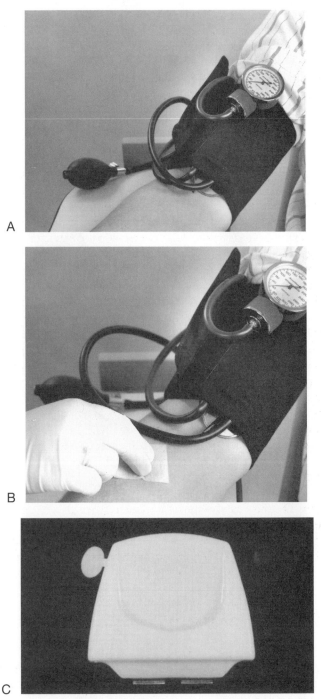

FIGURE 6-1 • *A*, Sphygmomanometer inflated to 40 mm Hg. *B*, Cleansing the site. *C*, Commercial bleeding-time instrument.

Illustration continued on following page

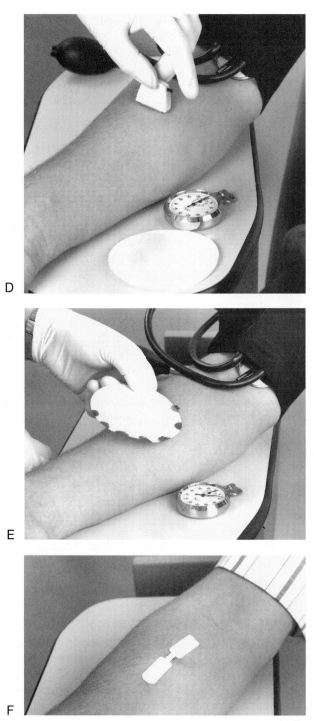

FIGURE 6-1 • *Continued*   *D,* Making the incision. *E,* Blotting. *F,* Butterfly bandage applied after bleeding stopped.

screening tests are for increased bilirubin, phenylketonuria (PKU) and hypothyroidism, the latter two required by law in the U.S.A. Bilirubin is a screen for hemolytic disease of the newborn and PKU screens the infant for the ability to metabolize **phenylalanine.** Inability to metabolize phenylalanine can result in brain damage and mental retardation. Screening for hypothyroidism will detect if the thyroid gland is underperforming, which can result in a general slowing of many functions.

Collecting blood from infants involves using a variation of the microcollection techniques previously discussed in Chapter 5. The site of collection is generally the infant's foot. Care must be exercised when performing the skin puncture to avoid damaging the heel bone, which can cause **osteomyelitis** in the newborn. Figure 6–2A illustrates the safe areas to perform the puncture.

When preparing to perform the blood collection, take only the equipment necessary into the bassinet area to avoid needlessly exposing a generally weakened infant to additional bacteria. You will usually be required to wear at least a gown in addition to gloves. Try not to disturb the infant any more than necessary, and if you must change the infant's position, do so only with permission of the nurse because of the many tubes and lines that are often attached to premature infants. Prepare the puncture site as described in Chapter 5, and hold the heel firmly as shown in Figure 6–2B. Perform the skin puncture and wipe away the first drop of blood. Collect blood into the appropriate container, being careful not to apply too much pressure to the heel; this could adversely affect the results of testing, as well as hurt the infant. When you are finished, apply pressure until bleeding has stopped. *Do not apply a bandage, and do not leave anything in the bassinet.* Label the collected specimens appropriately and deliver them to the laboratory. The collection for the PKU and hypothyroidism involves blotting of the infant's blood on specially prepared testing paper. As with all procedures, carefully read instructions.

Because of the small total blood volume of newborns (Fig. 6–3), a log should be kept of the total blood removed from infants. Often anemia becomes a problem because of the amount of blood collected from a given newborn. Therefore, accurate records must be maintained.

SYRINGE COLLECTIONS

At one time a syringe was the only option for blood collection. With the advent of the evacuated tube system, the use of a syringe to collect venous blood is no longer routine. Generally, a syringe is used to collect blood from veins that may collapse when using an evacuated tube system due to the force of the vacuum (e.g., small or fragile veins often found in elderly patients and small children). See Figure 6–4 for an illustration of a typical syringe.

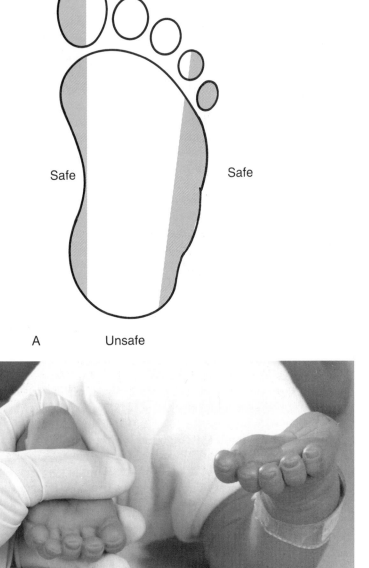

FIGURE 6-2 • *A*, Safe areas on an infant's foot for microcapillary collection. *B*, A properly held heel for skin puncture.

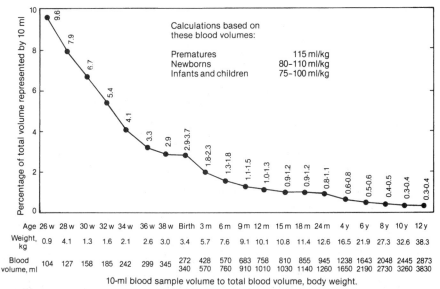

Calculations based on these blood volumes:

Prematures	115 ml/kg
Newborns	80–110 ml/kg
Infants and children	75–100 ml/kg

Age	26 w	28 w	30 w	32 w	34 w	36 w	38 w	Birth	3 m	6 m	9 m	12 m	15 m	18 m	24 m	4 y	6 y	8 y	10 y	12 y
Weight, kg	0.9	4.1	1.3	1.6	2.1	2.6	3.0	3.4	5.7	7.6	9.1	10.1	10.8	11.4	12.6	16.5	21.9	27.3	32.6	38.3
Blood volume, ml	104	127	158	185	242	299	345	272 340	428 570	570 760	683 910	758 1010	810 1030	855 1140	945 1260	1238 1650	1643 2190	2048 2730	2445 3260	2873 3830

10-ml blood sample volume to total blood volume, body weight.

FIGURE 6-3 • Relationship of 10 mL blood sample to total blood volume, body weight, and age of patient. (From Stockbower JM, Blumenfeld TA. eds. Collection and handling of laboratory specimens. Philadelphia, Lippincott, 1983.)

Collecting blood via the syringe is really rather simple. Preparation of the venipuncture site is the same as that for the evacuated tube system described in Chapter 5. However, use of the syringe does differ significantly from that of the evacuated tube system in the order in which the tubes are filled once the blood is collected in the syringe. Because blood will begin to clot in the syringe, it is imperative that collected blood be added to the anticoagulant tubes (i.e., the sodium citrate [blue-stoppered] tubes) first, followed by any other anticoagulant tubes, and then any remaining tubes without anticoagulant. The phlebotomist should mix the anticoagulant tubes thoroughly after the blood has been added, and it is advisable to carefully remove the syringe needle to facilitate the addition of blood to the tubes. Figure 6–5 illustrates the order for tube filling. When adding the blood, do not "squirt" the blood in the tubes but rather

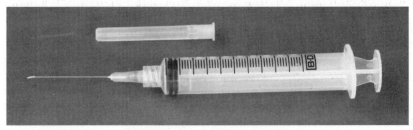

FIGURE 6-4 • A typical syringe.

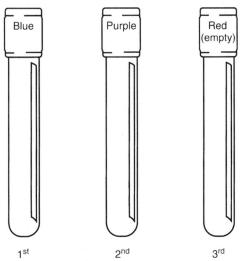

FIGURE 6-5 • Proper order for filling tubes with blood collected via syringe. Sodium citrate anticoagulant tubes (blue-stoppered) must be filled first, followed by any other anticoagulant tubes and then any remaining tubes without anticoagulant.

allow the blood to steadily flow down the sides of the tubes. In this manner, hemolysis may be avoided.

GLUCOSE TOLERANCE TEST

The glucose tolerance test (GTT) is done on individuals who are being screened for **diabetes mellitus** or **hypoglycemia.** The purpose of the test is to determine the patient's blood glucose level after the patient consumes a fixed amount of glucose (usually 100 gm). The test takes from 3 to 5 hours. Although there is nothing unique about the actual collection process itself, the number of venipunctures performed in a relatively short period of time make this test significant.

After a patient has fasted for at least 12 hours, a blood sample is collected using routine collection procedures. The blood may be collected in a plain tube (without any anticoagulant) or in a tube especially designed to preserve glucose levels (e.g., gray-stoppered tubes with sodium fluoride and potassium oxalate).

After the fasting sample is collected, the patient is directed to consume 100 gm of glucose as quickly as possible, often in liquid form. *It is critical to note the time of glucose consumption and of all subsequent venipunctures.* Blood is then collected at ½ hour, 1 hour, 2 hours, 3 hours, etc., up to 5 hours after consuming the glucose. At each venipuncture a urine specimen is also collected. Again, it is very important to note the collection time on all specimens. The procedure may terminate in less than 5 hours depending upon local protocol.

The laboratory analyzes the glucose levels in the blood specimens and plots them on a chart (Fig. 6–6). The results help the physician determine whether the patient is suffering from diabetes.

The phlebotomist plays a very crucial role in the administration of this test. Usually the patient receives a set of instructions about what to eat and a warning to avoid stressful exercise in the days leading up to the GTT. However, it is often the phlebotomist who gives the patient instructions about dieting and fasting. The patient should eat a well-balanced diet for 3 days before the test. Generally, the patient is allowed water and is actually encouraged to drink water during the fast and the test, but nothing else is allowed, including coffee and tea. Smoking is also

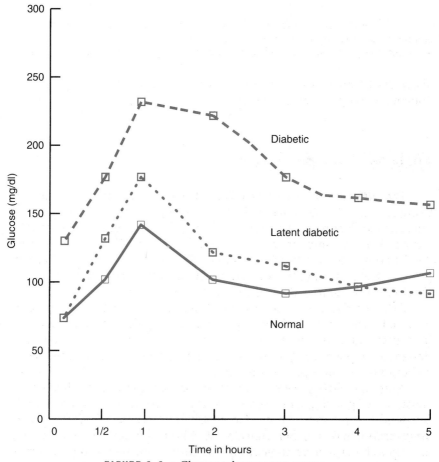

FIGURE 6-6 • Glucose tolerance test curves.

discouraged. These instructions must be delivered in a clear and understandable manner. Patients should be encouraged to ask questions if they do not understand the instructions. If the phlebotomist does not perform this patient education function properly, much valuable time may be wasted.

Finally, the phlebotomist must be prepared to handle the situation when the patient becomes ill from consuming the glucose or "lightheaded" from fasting for several hours. Sometimes, nausea and vomiting occur early in the test, and it is a good idea to have towels and an emesis basin nearby. If the patient vomits within the first ½ hour, the test should be discontinued and will probably need to be rescheduled for another day. It would be appropriate to notify the patient's physician and have him or her make the final decision. If the patient vomits or becomes faint later in the test, have him or her lie down, and complete the testing. If repeated oral glucose administrations are unsuccessful, intravenously administered glucose is an option. The patient's physician will make this decision.

ARTERIAL PUNCTURES

Although they are *very infrequently* performed by phlebotomists, arterial punctures should be mentioned. Generally, a nurse or respiratory therapist will collect an arterial blood specimen to assay for blood gases. The blood gas determination reveals, among other things, how well the lungs are functioning in terms of gas exchange. It should be clearly explained to the patient that this procedure is more uncomfortable than venipuncture and more difficult to accomplish.

The obvious difference between the arterial puncture and the venipuncture is the blood vessel from which the specimen is collected. The artery of choice is often the brachial artery, which is located on the inside of the upper arm (Fig. 6–7). It can be found by feeling for a pulse using the middle finger and forefinger; the thumb is not used because its pulse may be confused with that of the artery. A second possible site is the radial artery found in the wrist area.

The puncture site should be cleansed with a provodine-iodine (Betadine) solution. No tourniquet is needed because of the pressure that already exists within the arteries. A syringe may be used, since generally only a small amount of blood (1 ml) is needed. The angle of entry is generally 45 degrees or greater. The syringe should be capped, placed in ice, and transported to the laboratory as soon as possible after collection. Ideally, the test should be run within 10 minutes after collection.

The phlebotomist should maintain pressure on the site for at least 15 minutes after collection. It takes much longer for bleeding to stop in an artery than in a vein. The patient should never be allowed to maintain pressure, and the patient's nurse should be made aware that

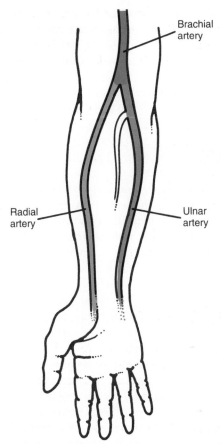

FIGURE 6-7 • The brachial artery is the preferred site for arterial puncture. A wrist artery may also be used.

an arterial puncture was done so that she or he can periodically check the puncture site.

COLD AGGLUTININ TESTS

A cold agglutinin is an antibody that is made in response to a form of pneumonia called primary atypical pneumonia, which is caused by the bacteria *Mycoplasma pneumoniae*. Therefore, the presence of a cold agglutinin is diagnostic. Occasionally the antibody can cause a form of autoimmune hemolytic anemia.

The key to collection of a specimen that will be screened for cold agglutinins is maintaining the specimen at 37°C after collection. The specimen is collected in an empty evacuated tube (plain red stopper) after proper site preparation and delivered promptly to the laboratory, where it is placed in a 37°C incubator at which temperature the blood must clot. If prompt delivery is not possible, the specimen may be placed in a temporary holding device such as a cup of water that is 37°C. The water must not be warmer than 37°C, as this may alter the test result. Similarly, should the specimen be allowed to cool, the results may be invalid.

BLOOD CULTURES

Under normal conditions, blood is a sterile substance. When bacteria enter into the bloodstream, this condition is referred to as **septicemia.** Septicemia is a very serious condition and must be detected and treated as soon as possible. Because blood circulates throughout the body, bacteria in the blood can be transported to other areas of the body, thereby spreading infection. The proper antibiotics must be administered to stop the infection.

To administer the proper antibiotics, the offending bacteria must be identified. To do this, a blood culture must be performed. The phlebotomist's role is to collect a specimen using special sterilization techniques.

One symptom of septicemia is a fever of unknown origin (FUO). Often such a fever will rise and fall on a regular basis. Therefore, timing of the blood culture is crucial. It is often desirable to collect blood cultures before and after a fever "spikes." This maximizes the chances of collecting a specimen while the bacteria is present in the bloodstream.

After a vein is located, the site is specially prepared for venipuncture. With the tourniquet off, the site is thoroughly scrubbed using surgical green soap for 2 minutes. A sterile alcohol pad is used to remove the soap by rubbing in outward-moving concentric circles (Fig. 6–8). The alcohol must be allowed to air dry. The site is then cleaned with a povidone-iodine solution, which is also allowed to air dry. The tourniquet is

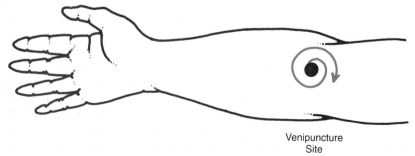

Venipuncture
Site

FIGURE 6-8 • Proper method for swabbing a venipuncture site, moving in an outward spiral.

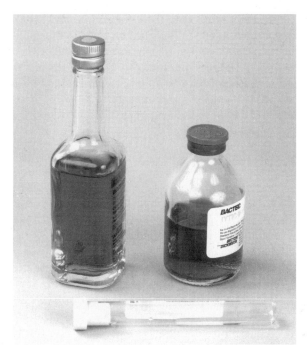

FIGURE 6-9 • Examples of culture systems used in collection of blood cultures. *Left*, specially designed vacutainer tube for collecting a blood culture (direct method). *Right*, typical blood culture bottle (indirect method). *Front*, vacuum tube (yellow-top) for collecting blood cultures.

applied, and the venipuncture is performed. The site can be touched only with sterile gauze or with a finger that has been cleaned in the same way used for the site.

Although some aspects of blood culture collection will vary from institution to institution, all techniques involve collecting blood either directly or indirectly into an **aerobic** and **anaerobic** culture system. Either a syringe or a specially designed evacuated tube is used (Fig. 6–9 left). When a syringe is used, a clean needle is placed on the syringe after blood collection to avoid possible contamination, and then the blood culture bottles are inoculated (anaerobic followed by aerobic).

The blood may also be collected into an evacuated tube made especially for blood cultures. (Fig. 6–9 Front.) This is usually a yellow-stoppered tube with sodium polyanethol sulfonate (SPS) which prevents coagulation and inhibits complement and phagocytosis. Then, in the laboratory, a syringe is used to remove blood from the evacuated tube and inoculate the blood culture bottles (Fig. 6–9 Right). However, no matter what collection method is used, care must be taken to maintain sterility by swabbing the septum of the culture bottles with iodine followed by alcohol.

After the blood is collected, the povidone-iodine solution can be removed using alcohol swabs. The culture bottles must be thoroughly mixed and labeled with pertinent information, including the time and site of collection. This is important, because blood cultures are collected rather frequently, and the policy at some hospitals is to alternate arms at each blood culture collection.

BLOOD DONATION COLLECTIONS

Phlebotomists may be employed in a blood donation center, where they collect blood that will ultimately be used for transfusion. These centers may be American Red Cross Centers, Community Blood Centers, or hospital blood banks and collection centers.

Phlebotomists who collect blood from volunteer donors must be very competent in the skill of venipuncture and must possess good interpersonal skills. Because relatively few individuals (less than 5% of the population) provide donor blood for the entire country, it is very critical that every phase of the donation process be performed smoothly and professionally. The health care system cannot afford the loss of these volunteer donors, and an unpleasant experience may discourage them from volunteering again.

This type of blood collection varies from routine venipuncture in two ways: the amount of blood that is collected (usually 450 ml) and the nature of the "patient." Individuals who donate blood must undergo a thorough medical history and screening. The history should include frequency of donation, present and past medications, exposure to transfusion-transmitted disease such as hepatitis B and human immuno-deficiency virus (HIV), recent vaccinations, foreign travel, and cancer history. The medical screening includes monitoring blood pressure, temperature, hemoglobin or hematocrit, weight, pulse, skin lesions, and general appearance. Donors also complete a donor self-exclusion form, which allows them to confidentially ensure that their blood will not be used for transfusion if they have any misgivings. The American Association of Blood Banks' *Technical Manual* contains a more thorough discussion of donor criteria. Once the donor passes the medical history and screening, the actual phlebotomy can be performed. The antecubital area of the arm is the preferred site and must be thoroughly cleaned and disinfected. (See the procedure discussed earlier for blood culture preparation.) The step-by-step procedure for performing blood donor phlebotomy is as follows:

1. Once the donor is comfortably situated—generally on a bed or special donor chair—locate the vein.

2. Prepare the site.

3. Prepare the blood collection bag and scale. Be sure there is a clamp between the bag and the needle.

4. Apply the tourniquet or blood pressure cuff (inflated to 40 to 60 mm Hg), and give the donor something to squeeze. These techniques will help distend the vein.

5. Perform the venipuncture and place the needle approximately ½ inch into the vein.

6. Release the clamp; if there is a steady flow of blood into the bag, tape the needle to the arm. Cover the area with sterile gauze.

7. Release the tourniquet or blood pressure cuff, but instruct the donor to clench his or her fist. Monitor the donor for any adverse reactions. (These are infrequent; see Chapter 7.)

8. When the appropriate volume of blood (405 to 450 ml) is collected, instruct the donor to stop clenching the fist, and clamp or tie a knot in the tubing.

9. Collect pilot tubes—samples of donor blood that will be tested before the unit is released for transfusion—before removing the needle from the donor's arm.

10. Strip the tubing and thoroughly mix the blood; then allow the tubing to refill. At this time the tubing may be segmented.

11. Place the units in storage as specified by the collection room nurse or technologist.

12. Do not allow the patient to arise or leave the area until bleeding has stopped and at least 10 minutes have elapsed. Because the donor has lost a significant amount of blood, be sure to instruct him or her to increase fluid intake over the next 24 hours, avoid alcohol until after a meal, avoid smoking for at least 30 minutes, refrain from strenuous exercise for a few hours, apply pressure if bleeding resumes, and sit down if dizziness occurs. They may have to return to the blood bank or see their own doctor if symptoms continue.

13. Finally, *always be polite and professional.* The donor should leave with a positive feeling so that he or she will be inclined to donate blood again.

THERAPEUTIC COLLECTIONS

As mentioned in Chapter 1, in ancient times, therapeutic phlebotomy was the only treatment used for many different conditions. Today the treatment is used very judiciously. Blood is collected as an aid to treatment of some diseases such as **polycythemia vera** or **myasthenia gravis.** It is rarely the definitive treatment, but instead serves as symptomatic treatment until the underlying cause can be identified and treated.

Therapeutic phlebotomies are very similar to donor blood collection, but the underlying purpose is different. Whereas donated blood is destined to be used for transfusion, blood collected for a therapeutic reason is generally discarded or occasionally is used for research purposes. Therefore, no additional pilot tubes of blood need be collected for additional testing. In addition, the amount of blood collected may be different; an amount less than 450 ml may be appropriate depending on the patient's age and condition. However, site preparation is the same, and the same precautions must be observed when performing therapeutic phlebotomies.

TESTS FOR FIBRIN DEGRADATION PRODUCTS

Fibrin degradation products (FDPs) are the result of the disintegration of fibrin or fibrinogen by plasmin, a coagulation enzyme. Increased levels of FDPs are generally associated with such conditions as myocardial infarctions, pulmonary emboli, certain complications of pregnancy, and disseminated intravascular coagulation.

A popular test for detecting FDPs is the Thrombo–Wellcotest (Burroughs–Wellcome, Triangle Park, NC). For the phlebotomist, this test involves performing a routine venipuncture using a tube provided with the test kit. The tube will hold 2 ml of blood and contains a special enzyme inhibitor plus thrombin. It is important to avoid traumatic venipunctures that might result in hemolysis, and the sample must be gently but thoroughly mixed after collection. Additionally, it must be allowed to stand for 15 minutes before any centrifugation.

Once the sample is collected, assays are performed in the laboratory to semiquantitate the FDPs. This information is important to the clinician in making the proper diagnosis. Occasionally, urine may be tested for FDPs.

PERIPHERAL BLOOD SMEARS

Peripheral blood smears are important to the clinician for a number of reasons. Examination of the blood smear may reveal abnormal red cell morphology characteristic of certain disease states such as sickle cell anemia (Fig. 6–10). The variety and proportion of white blood cells may also be ascertained; information of this nature may also help in the diagnosis of disease. For example, infectious mononucleosis is characterized by an increased number of "atypical" lymphocytes.

Although the process is becoming increasingly semiautomated, phlebotomists may still be called on to make a blood smear. This may be done either at the patient's bedside using standard microscope slides and capillary blood or in the laboratory using well-mixed, recently collected (within 1 hour) anticoagulated (with ethylenediaminetetra-acetate) blood.

The "wedge" method is probably the most common manual method (Fig. 6–11). The following important points should be remembered:

- Keep the smear slide on a flat surface.
- Make the smear immediately after placing the blood on the slide.
- Make the smear in a smooth fashion to avoid ridges and bubbles.
- Allow the smear to air dry; never blow on it.
- A straight-edge smear is preferable to a bullet-shaped smear because of better distribution of leukocytes.

It takes a great deal of practice to become proficient at making smears, and therefore it may be desirable to assign slide making to certain members of the phlebotomy team.

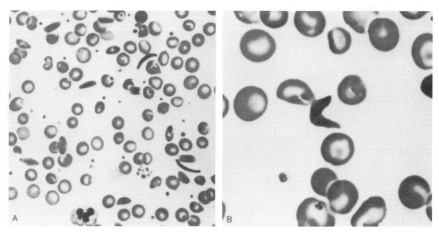

FIGURE 6-10 • Blood smear from a patient with sickle cell anemia. *A,* Low magnification shows sickled cells. *B,* Higher magnification shows an irreversible sickled cell in the center. (Courtesy of Dr. Robert W. McKenna, University of Texas, Southwestern Medical School, Dallas, TX)

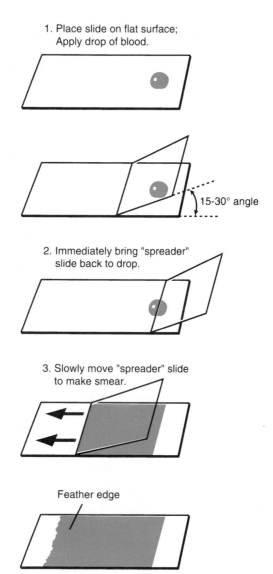

1. Place slide on flat surface; Apply drop of blood.

15-30° angle

2. Immediately bring "spreader" slide back to drop.

3. Slowly move "spreader" slide to make smear.

Feather edge

FIGURE 6-11 • "Wedge" method, the suggested method for making blood smears.

REVIEW QUESTIONS

1. Arterial puncture is the method of choice for

   _____ .

2. The volume of blood usually collected during

   blood donation is _____ .

3. Bacteria in the blood is referred to as _____ .

4. _____ is an infection of the bone
   that may be caused by penetration of the heel
   bone with a lancet.

5. The device inflated to 40 mm Hg when a phlebotomist is performing the Ivy bleeding time

   test is a _____ .

6. _____ and _____ are neonatal
   tests required by law.

7. The _____ is used to test patients for
   diabetes mellitus and hypoglycemia.

8. Sodium polyanethol sulfonate is an additive in

   _____ stoppered tubes.

Bibliography

Goss CM, ed. Gray's Anatomy: Anatomy of the human body (28th ed.). Philadelphia, Lea & Febiger, 1966.

Harmening DM, ed. Clinical hematology and fundamentals of hemostasis (3rd ed.). Philadelphia, FA Davis, 1997.

Nursing79 Books. (1978). Managing Diabetics Properly. Horsham, PA: Intermed Communications Inc.

Slockbower JM, Blumenfeld TA, eds. Collection and handling of laboratory specimens, Philadelphia, Lippincott, 1983.

Tietz NW, ed. Fundamentals of clinical chemistry (3rd ed.). Philadelphia, Saunders, 1987.

Walker RH, ed. Technical manual (11th ed.). Arlington, VA, American Association of Blood Banks, 1993.

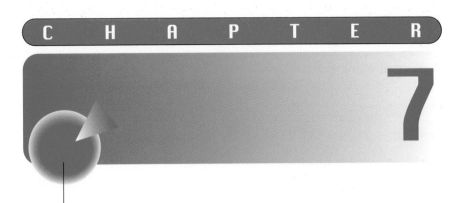

7

Complications of Phlebotomy

John C. Flynn, Jr.

135

This chapter will discuss various complications that can be encountered while performing or attempting to perform phlebotomy. These include uncooperative or absent patients, medical/physiologic complications, and technical problems.

THE UNCOOPERATIVE PATIENT

Every phlebotomist has encountered an uncooperative patient. The patient may be uncooperative for a variety of reasons such as age [young or old], which may preclude him or her from understanding the procedure; there may be mental dysfunction; or the patient may object to having the phlebotomy done for some other reason.

When a patient is too old or young to understand what is going on and will probably resist or struggle, do not attempt to perform the venipuncture alone. Get help from the patient's nurse, a fellow phlebotomist, or a parent, relative, or guardian. Take precautions to ensure the safety of the individual, but do not compromise your own safety. A common and safe way to hold a child is shown in Figure 7–1A and B.

Occasionally phlebotomists are required to collect blood from a patient who is mentally disturbed, mentally retarded, or suffering from substance abuse. In such a case, the patient may not understand the procedure and may react violently. You must do what you can to reassure the patient and secure cooperation. However, if there is any doubt about how the patient will react, do not attempt to collect the specimen until you have secured some assistance, even if the patient is in restraints.

Sometimes a patient may be of sound mind and yet still refuse to have the procedure performed. At these times you must use your skills of persuasion to convince the patient to allow you to collect the blood sample. Point out that the physician needs the blood test results to properly manage the patient's illness and prescribe the proper medication. Never attempt to force, either physically or with threats, a patient in this situation. A patient has the right to refuse a blood draw. Ultimately, if the patient refuses to allow the blood collection, this must be noted on the requisition form, which is returned to the laboratory; the patient's nurse must also be informed.

Another situation that often confronts a phlebotomist is that of an absent patient—that is, the patient is not where he or she is supposed to be. The patient may have been moved to another room or transported to surgery or the radiology department. He or she may have been discharged or perhaps may have **expired.** Generally, the phlebotomist can find out where the patient is by asking the nurse in charge. If the patient

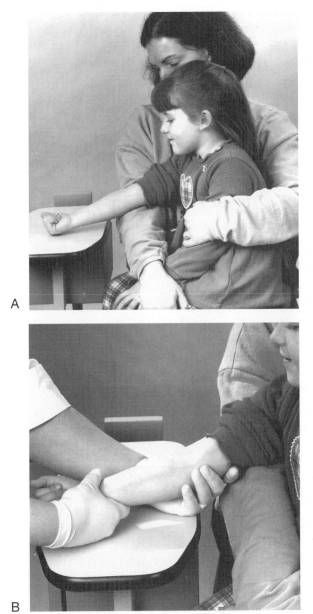

FIGURE 7-1 • *A* and *B*, A suggested way to restrain a child for phlebotomy.

has simply been moved to another room, collect the blood specimen, noting the room change on the requisition form and on the tube of blood. If the patient is inaccessible (e.g., in radiology or the operating room), inform the patient's nurse and note on the requisition form why the blood was not collected.

MEDICAL/PHYSIOLOGIC COMPLICATIONS

COMMON COMPLICATIONS

Syncope

Syncope, more commonly referred to as fainting, results from insufficient blood flow to the brain. This can be caused by fatigue, a sudden decrease in blood volume, cardiac arrhythmia, hypoglycemia, or hyperventilation. However, fainting is primarily due to psychological causes in individuals who are having their blood collected. Merely the sight of blood or needles is enough to cause some people to faint.

To prevent fainting or to deal effectively with it, the phlebotomist must always be aware of the condition of the patient. Observe the patient before the phlebotomy; is he or she acting nervous or hyperventilating? Try to engage the patient in conversation to keep his or her mind off the procedure. After performing the venipuncture, ask the patient how he or she feels.

Whereas the volume of blood collected during routine phlebotomy is not enough in itself to cause fainting due to **hypovolemia,** hypovolemia may cause fainting in blood donation. As stated in Chapter 6, blood donation results in about a 450-ml loss of blood from the donor. This loss may be enough to cause syncope if the patient attempts to get out of the donor chair/table too quickly. For this reason, the donor is not allowed to leave the chair for at least 10 minutes after the collection. This time, along with the consumption of some liquids, gives the body a chance to adjust to the decreased total blood volume.

If a patient is sitting in a phlebotomy chair and faints before the venipuncture, put the patient's head between his or her knees (Fig. 7–2). A cold compress placed on the back of the neck is also helpful. It is also a good idea to have ammonium salts available, but these can be very strong and must be used with care. Once the patient recovers, have him or her lie down for the phlebotomy to be performed. A cool drink may also help the patient feel better. Patients who are lying down very seldom feel faint. If the patient feels faint after the phlebotomy has been started, remove the tourniquet, carefully remove the needle, and, while applying pressure, support the patient and call for help. *Never leave the patient!*

Hematoma

Probably the most common complication from phlebotomy is the **hematoma.** This occurs when the needle is improperly placed in the vein, allowing blood to escape from the vein and collect under the skin (Fig.

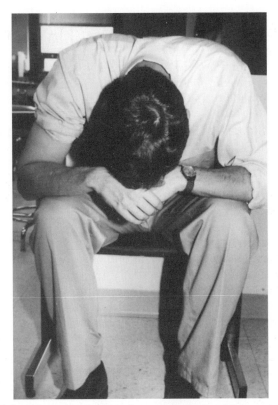

FIGURE 7-2 • If the patient feels faint, place the head between the knees.

7–3). The primary indication of a hematoma is swelling around the venipuncture site while the needle is inserted. By adjusting the depth of the needle, it may be possible to stop the hematoma from enlarging. Otherwise, remove the needle and apply firm pressure to the site. This may help the blood to disperse somewhat. It is usually good practice and

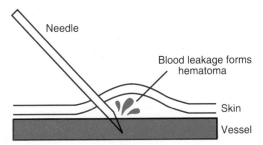

FIGURE 7-3 • A hematoma occurs when an improperly placed needle causes blood to escape from the vein.

common courtesy to inform the patient that he or she may notice a bruise in a day or two at the venipuncture site. It is nothing to be alarmed about and will disappear in a few days.

If removal of the needle is required and not enough blood was collected, another venipuncture must be performed. This venipuncture should be at an alternate site.

Hematomas may occur after the phlebotomy is completed. This is why it is very important to maintain pressure on the venipuncture site until bleeding has stopped.

SHORT DRAW OR NO BLOOD COLLECTED

Occasionally, the phlebotomist will enter the vein, and the blood flow will be slow, stop after a short time, or will not flow at all. There are some general technical errors that can occur; these are discussed later. There are also some occasions when the needle is in the vein, but blood flow is reduced. In such cases, the needle bevel may be against the vessel wall, thus preventing the flow of blood. Slight manipulation of the needle will generally remedy this problem. In other cases the suction of the tube vacuum may be too great, causing the vessel to collapse (Fig. 7–4). In these cases smaller tubes or a syringe may be used to collect the blood. Collapsed veins may also occur if the syringe plunger is withdrawn too quickly.

Another cause of insufficient collection may occur when the needle is not inserted far enough. The needle may be below the skin surface, but above the vein. Gently inserting the needle into the vein should result in blood flow. Conversely, the needle may have been inserted through the vein, thus no blood collected. Slowly withdrawing the needle back into the vein will correct this problem. See Figure 7–5.

Finally, it should be noted that anticoagulated tubes, i.e., blue, lavender, etc., must be filled to the proper level. Short-draws in these tubes will alter the anticoagulant to blood ratio resulting in spurious results. Nonanticoagulated tubes, i.e., red tops and speckled tops, may be used if a short-draw occurs.

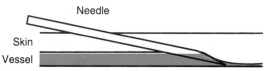

FIGURE 7-4 • One possible cause of a "short draw," or failure to obtain blood. The vacuum causes the vessel to collapse.

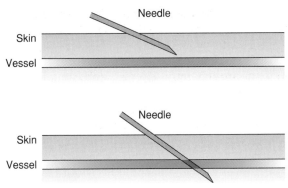

FIGURE 7-5 • Possible explanations for not collecting blood. In the top picture, the needle is not inserted deeply enough. In the bottom picture, the needle is inserted too deeply.

LESS COMMON COMPLICATIONS

Petechiae. Petechiae are small red dots that appear on the skin as the result of capillary **hemorrhage.** In such cases, the capillaries bleed excessively because of a coagulation problem, generally one related to platelets. As stated in Chapter 2, the function of platelets is to stop bleeding from blood vessel walls. If you notice petechiae, you should realize that it may take a little longer than normal for the patient to stop bleeding from the venipuncture site. Petechiae can also be the result of tying the tourniquet too tight and leaving it on too long. For this reason the tourniquet should not be on for longer than 1 to 2 minutes.

Edema. Edema results when excessive fluids collect in the tissues of a patient, resulting in swelling. Venipuncture should be avoided in these areas, because (1) it is often difficult to locate a vein, and (2) the specimen may be diluted with tissue fluids, which could adversely affect the testing results.

Excessive Bleeding. A phlebotomist must not leave a patient until bleeding has stopped following venipuncture. Normally, this is a few minutes. However, occasionally patients on anticoagulant therapy may take much longer. It is the phlebotomist's responsibility to be certain that bleeding has stopped.

IV Lines. Phlebotomy should be avoided from an area adjacent to or above an intravenous (IV) line. Use the arm without the IV or some other site. If a phlebotomy must be collected from the arm with the IV, draw the blood from below the IV. If blood is drawn above the IV, the IV should be stopped and a note sent to the laboratory indicating that the blood was collected above an IV. Be sure to check local protocol with respect to collecting blood above an IV.

Obesity. Locating and palpating a vein may be difficult in an obese patient, as the veins are generally "deeper" and cannot be seen. However, with practice and patience, you will learn to locate these veins and perform the phlebotomy with minimal difficulty.

Allergies. Occasionally patients may indicate that they are allergic to a sterilizing solution or to the adhesive on bandages. When a patient expresses these concerns, the phlebotomist should find an alternative.

Damaged or Scarred Ueins. Occasionally you will encounter a patient who has had so many venipunctures that an area of scar tissue has developed around the area that you plan to use for phlebotomy. For example, it is not unusual for intravenous drug users to have a lot of scar tissue. These situations require an alternative site for venipuncture, and if none can be located (which would be unusual), a microcapillary procedure should be considered. Veins may also be damaged or occluded (blocked) to the degree that even if the venipuncture is successful, little blood is collected. Again, an alternate site must be located.

Burned Areas. Burned areas must be avoided altogether, as they are very susceptible to infection. The phlebotomist must take extra precautions when performing venipuncture on these patients. Gowns and face masks are required, because the patient is at risk of contracting an infection from the phlebotomist (see Chap. 3). An alternate site for venipuncture must be chosen or a microcollection technique utilized.

Conuulsions. Although **convulsions** resulting from phlebotomy are rare, a phlebotomist must be prepared to deal with them. It is a good practice to ask patients if they have had any previous adverse reactions to phlebotomy. Although many things can cause convulsions, simple hysteria causes most convulsions in phlebotomy patients. The most important thing is to not let patients harm themselves. If the needle is in the arm, quickly remove it and the tourniquet, if the latter is still on the arm. Move anything that could harm the patient and try to protect the patient's head from striking an object that could cause harm. Do not forget to call for help and notify a physician. If the patient is in a phlebotomy chair and starts to fall out, help guide him or her to the floor. *Do not panic, and never leave the patient alone!* Be sure to record the date, time, and circumstances under which the convulsion occurred. Once the patient recovers, assess the situation to determine whether the phlebotomy can be done or repeated, if required, or whether the patient should return at a later time. Finally, the supervisor of the phlebotomy team or unit must be notified.

Mastectomy. Venipuncture should be avoided in the arm on the same side in which a **mastectomy** was performed. This is because the patient may be very susceptible to infection on that side of the body due to removal of lymph nodes concurrently with the breast. In the case of a double mastectomy, the patient's physician or nurse should be consulted.

TECHNICAL PROBLEMS

The technical problems discussed in this section include situations that result in no blood being collected because of either faulty equipment or simply missing the vein. Occasionally everything is done properly, but when the tube is pushed onto the needle, no blood is forthcoming. This could be due to a faulty collection tube that does not contain any vacuum or because the phlebotomist unknowingly pushed the tube onto the needle during the process of preparing to perform the venipuncture, thus releasing the vacuum. It is always a good practice to carry extra collection tubes and keep them within easy reach whenever performing a phlebotomy.

Another technical problem that occasionally occurs is having the needle unscrew from the barrel during the phlebotomy. If this occurs, do not attempt to correct the problem; simply discontinue the phlebotomy, and repeat the procedure. Make sure that the needle is properly seated in the hub of the barrel so that the problem does not happen again, and the needle cover is pulled and not twisted when being removed.

All phlebotomists, at some point in their career, will miss the target vein completely. When this occurs, it may be possible to simply redirect the needle slightly and obtain blood. You may be to one side of the vein or perhaps did not enter the needle deep enough. *However, avoid probing!* The more experience you get as a phlebotomist, the less frequently you will miss, and when you do, it will be easier for you to redirect the needle without having to repeat the entire venipuncture procedure.

SPECIMEN REJECTION

This section will outline some of the common reasons why specimens may be rejected by the clinical laboratory.

HEMOLYSIS

Hemolysis occurs when red blood cells are destroyed, thus releasing a red-tinted substance, hemoglobin. Hemolysis may not be evident at the time of collection but becomes evident in the laboratory when the specimens are centrifuged to separate the cells from the serum or plasma.

TABLE 7-1 • The Effects of Hemolysis on Common Tests

Test	Effect
Chemistry	
Potassium	Increased value
Magnesium	Increased value
Aldolase	Increased value
Lactate dehydrogenase	Increased value
Blood bank	
Antibody screen	May invalidate test; specimen rejected
Hematology	
Prothrombin time	Increased value if severe
Activated partial thromboplastin time	Increased value if severe

The serum or plasma will have a pink/red tint. The greater the hemolysis, the more color will be present and the more laboratory test results may be affected. Depending on the test being performed, a hemolyzed specimen may not be acceptable. For example, hemolysis may interfere with testing done in the blood bank. In other areas, the hemolysis or hemoglobin itself may not be a problem, but other constituents released when the cells were destroyed may interfere with testing or give falsely high or low values. See Table 7–1 for some common tests and the effect hemolysis may have on them.

Hemolysis may be a result of a physiologic condition, such as autoimmune hemolytic anemia or a transfusion reaction, that causes hemoglobin to be present in the patient's plasma. More often it is a result of the venipuncture procedure itself or the handling of the specimen after collection. See Table 7–2 for a list of items that may result in a specimen being hemolyzed.

TABLE 7-2 • Causes of Hemolysis

Technical
  Vigorously shaking the tube of blood
  Using a needle that is too small
  Drawing too hard on the syringe plunger
  Expelling blood too quickly through the syringe into the collection tubes
  Allowing the specimen to overheat
Physiologic
  Transfusion reaction
  Autoimmune hemolytic anemia
  Paroxysmal nocturnal hemoglobinuria
  Disseminated intravascular coagulation

If the phlebotomist follows standard procedures and is conscientious, most cases of phlebotomy-induced hemolysis can be avoided. This in turn will save time, money, and, most important, the need to perform a repeat phlebotomy on the patient.

HEMOCONCENTRATION

Hemoconcentration occurs when the tourniquet is on for too long. It results in a "backing up" or concentration of blood at the venipuncture site. As the blood backs up, specimens collected from the area will have falsely elevated red and white cell counts. This may only be detected if prior laboratory results are available for comparisons. If prior laboratory results are available and if there is a significant change in the cell counts without adequate explanation, the latest specimen may be rejected and a new specimen requested.

CLOTS

Clot formation occurs when **coagulation factors** are activated. Normally, if no anticoagulants are present in the collection tube, these factors are activated almost immediately. When a clot forms in an anticoagulant specimen, generally the specimen will be rejected and a new one will have to be collected. When a clot begins to form in an anticoagulated tube, it usually indicates that the blood and anticoagulant are not in proper balance. If too little blood is collected, or if too much blood is added to an anticoagulant tube—as, for example, via a syringe—a clot may form. Therefore, whenever using an evacuated tube system, always fill the tube with the amount of blood indicated.

Clots may also be present when blood is collected into a syringe and not expelled soon enough into an anticoagulant tube. For this reason blood collected via a syringe is expressed into an anticoagulant tube, rather than an empty tube, first.

Finally, clots may form because the anticoagulant itself is not active or is not present in the proper quantity. The phlebotomist may not be aware of this, and therefore, it is very important to check the expiration date on the tubes. As long as they are in date, everything should be acceptable.

SHORT DRAW

A short draw is a specimen that does not contain enough blood. Depending on the tests being performed, a short draw may result in specimen rejection. A short draw may occur when the needle comes out of the vein, the vein collapses, or the vacuum was not sufficient to fill the tube. If the vein collapses, you will probably have to redraw the specimen from a different site or possibly use a syringe. If the needle came out of the vein and you can reinsert it, you will avoid a short draw. Otherwise the venipuncture may need to be repeated. Possibly the vacuum was not strong enough; in this case, the extra tubes you should be carrying will enable you to collect the specimen without needing to "restick" the patient.

CLERICAL DISCREPANCIES

Clerical discrepancies occur when the name on the requisition form does not match the name on the tube of blood. Depending on the institution and the laboratory department, there will be variations in how clerical discrepancies are handled. For example, a specimen with a slightly misspelled patient name may be acceptable for hematology if the patient's hospital number, room number, etc., are correct. However, for transfusion units or blood banks, which have the strictest requirements, the slightest deviation in name or hospital number may require collection of a new specimen. The reason should be obvious: a transfusion based on the results of an incorrectly labeled specimen could be fatal!

REVIEW QUESTIONS

1. Small red dots on the skin indicating a possible coagulation problem are _PETECHIAE_ .

2. Low blood volume is referred to as _HYPOVOLEMIA_.

3. _EDEMA_ is a condition in which fluid collects in the tissues and results in swelling.

4. _HEMOLYSIS_ is the destruction of red blood cells that results in the release of hemoglobin.

5. Blood that escapes from a blood vessel and collects under the skin may result in a _HEMATOMA_ .

6. Blood donors are not allowed to leave the donor chair for 10 minutes because of the possibility of _SYNCOPE_ .

7. In women, venipuncture should be avoided in the arm on the side of a _MASTECTOMY_ .

Bibliography

Thomas CL, ed. Taber's cyclopedic medical dictionary (18th ed.). Philadelphia, FA Davis, 1997.

Tietz NW, ed. Fundamentals of clinical chemistry (3rd ed.). Philadelphia, Saunders, 1987.

Walker RH, ed. Technical manual (11th ed.). Arlington, VA: American Association of Blood Banks, 1993.

Multiskilling for Phlebotomists

Joyce E. Hill

In today's age of diversity, sometimes being trained in just one skill is not enough. This is the era of **multiskilling,** being able to be proficient at more than one job. Phlebotomists are no exception to this. With their extensive patient contact, they are one of the more obvious medical professionals to become crosstrained in several different skills. These skills can include, but are not limited to, those listed in Table 8-1.

Crosstraining or multiskilling can mean different things to different people, but to many it means greater job security, better marketability and, sometimes, more pay. To the phlebotomist, crosstraining can mean a better chance of obtaining employment. Many hospitals today are doing away with their phlebotomy departments. They are keeping phlebotomists for outpatient blood collection, but in-house blood collections are often no longer in the hands of the laboratory. In an effort to cut down on the number of hospital personnel an in-house patient may see, many hospitals are consolidating jobs. As with nurses who are "assigned" four or five patients for care, patients are also being "assigned" to one of these multiskilled technicians. The terms used to describe these multiskilled technicians are as varied as their job descriptions. Job titles may include, but are not limited to, patient care technicians, patient care associates, laboratory associates, laboratory services technicians, allied health technicians—the list goes on.

Not only are these multiskilled phlebotomists found in the hospital, they can also be employed in a doctor's office or an off-site blood collection station. In a doctor's office there usually is not enough work (or money) to employ a phlebotomist only, but a phlebotomist with additional training can become an asset in such a situation.

CARDIOPULMONARY RESUSCITATION

There is one skill in which all phlebotomists and, in fact, all health care workers should be trained, and that is cardiopulmonary resuscitation (CPR). As a phlebotomist, there may be times when you are working on your own, and a medical emergency takes place with your patient. There is a critical period of time before medical help is obtained or arrives

---

TABLE 8-1 • Skills for Crosstraining Phlebotomists

- EKGs
- Arterial blood gases
- Point-of-care testing (POCT)
- CLIA '88 waived testing
- CPR
- Assessing vital signs

---

that is of the utmost importance to your patient and may be the difference between life and death. First aid training, and more specifically CPR, will give the phlebotomist the ability to remain calm, exercise good judgment, and administer care in an orderly manner.

CPR is a combination of artificial respiration and artificial circulation to maintain the transfer of oxygen to the lungs and to circulate blood-containing oxygen to the patient's brain. CPR should only be performed by certified personnel. Certification may be obtained by taking a course offered by the American Red Cross, local hospital, American Heart Association, or other approved certification sites. Once certified, a refresher course needs to be taken every two years to maintain certification.

A CPR-certified phlebotomist can often be a plus to a potential employer. Employers can avoid the loss of time for training. Many phlebotomy courses are now offering CPR certification as part of their curriculum.

VITAL SIGNS

Besides CPR training, another skill that would benefit a phlebotomist is the ability to record vital signs. Vital signs consist of temperature, pulse, respiration (TPR), and blood pressure (BP). These skills would be of benefit whether employed in a donor center, doctor's office, or a hospital department.

TEMPERATURE

Body temperature is maintained in a fairly constant range, through a balance of the heat produced in the body and the heat lost by the body. Heat is produced through voluntary and involuntary muscle contractions. It is also produced through the breakdown of nutrients in the cells known as cell metabolism.

The balance of heat production and heat loss is controlled by the **hypothalamus** gland in the brain. The hypothalamus allows the body temperature to fluctuate about 1° to 2° Fahrenheit (F) throughout the day.

The normal body temperature range is 97° to 99°F (36° to 37.2° Centigrade [C]), with the average being 98.6°F or 37°C. There are four major areas for measuring temperature: oral (mouth), rectal, axillary, and aural (ear). It is very important to record the temperature site, as each site has its own normal reading.

Taking the temperature orally is the most convenient and common method. There is a rich supply of blood under the tongue and this is where the thermometer should be placed. In order for the reading to be accurate, the patient must keep his or her mouth closed over the ther-mometer. The normal reading for an oral temperature is 98.6°F or 37°C.

The rectal temperature is the most accurate because there are very few factors that can affect the results. The rectum has a rich blood supply and is a very closed cavity. Taking a temperature rectally requires a special thermometer, one that has a rounded tip. Normal rectal reading is 99.6°F or 37.6°C.

Axillary temperature is the least accurate of the four methods. This area is subject to a lot of variables. Since it is an open area, one must make sure that no clothing is in the way and that the thermometer is not exposed to any air. Also, the thermometer must be kept in place for approximately 10 minutes in order to obtain an accurate reading. Normal axillary temperature is 97.6°F or 36.4°C.

Tympanic (ear) is the newest process for taking temperature. It does, however, require a special thermometer which is known as a tympanic thermometer. This type of thermometer detects the energy that is radiated from the body through the tympanic membrane. This membrane is located very close to the hypothalamus and shares the same blood supply. The temperature taken this way is very accurate and gives instant results (within one second) without causing any discomfort to the patient. See Figure 8–1 for an illustration of a variety of temperature-recording devices.

PULSE

Pulse can be defined as the beat of the heart as felt through the wall of an artery. It is produced by a wave of blood passing through the artery with each contraction of the heart. The pulse can be felt by compressing an artery that is close to the surface and has an underlying solid structure such as bone.

The most common pulse sites are the radial, brachial, and carotid arteries. However, other sites may be used to assess circulation to those areas. (See Figure 8–2). Pulse sites are also used as pressure points to control severe bleeding.

Individual pulse rates vary according to the patient's age, gender, activity level, medications, and emotional state. See Table 8–2 for average pulse rate by age group.

When taking a pulse rate, other characteristics—rhythm and volume of the pulse—are noted. Rhythm refers to the time interval between heart beats, a normal rhythm having the same time interval between beats. Arrhythmias, abnormal rhythms, are characterized by unequal or irregu-lar intervals between heart beats. These must be noted.

The volume of the pulse refers to the strength of the beat felt. It

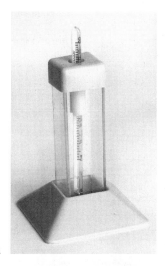

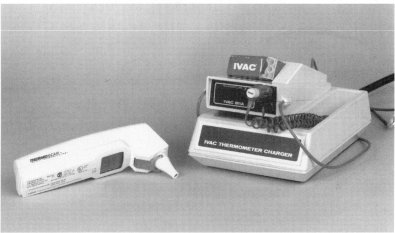

FIGURE 8-1 • Various models of thermometers: *A*, Standard oral thermometer. *B, (left)* Aural; *(right)* Variable site.

should feel full and strong, not weak and thready. Volume should also be noted.

RESPIRATION

Respiration is the act of breathing or the exchanging of gases: oxygen (O_2) and carbon dioxide (CO_2). One complete respiration consists of one inspiration or inhalation (taking air consisting of oxygen into the lungs) and one expiration or exhalation (expelling air containing carbon dioxide from the lungs).

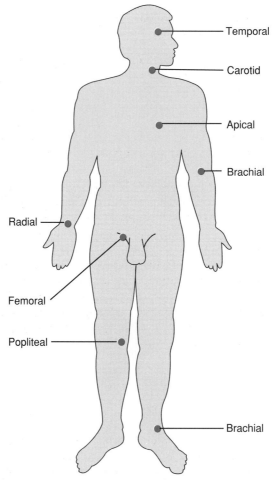

FIGURE 8-2 • Pulse sites.

Respiration can be further broken down into external and internal. External respiration is the exchange of oxygen and carbon dioxide taking place in the lungs between the alveoli and the blood. Internal respiration is the exchange of oxygen and carbon dioxide between the body cells and the blood.

TABLE 8-2 • Average Pulse Rate

Birth	130–160 beats/minute
Infants	110–130 beats/minute
Children (1–7 years)	80–120 beats/minute
Children over 7 years	80–90 beats/minute
Adults	60–80 beats/minute

TABLE 8-3 • Normal Respiration Rates

Infants	30–60 respirations/minute
Children (1–7 years)	18–30 respirations/minute
Adults	12–20 respirations/minute

Breathing is an involuntary act controlled by the medulla oblongata in the brain. To a point, a person holding his or her breath can also make breathing a voluntary act.

Characteristics of respiration include rate, rhythm, and depth. Respiratory rate is the number of respirations per minute. See Table 8-3.

There is a ratio of 1:4 respirations to a pulse. As with pulse rates, there are a wide variety of factors that will affect the respiratory rate. Some of these factors include age, physical activity, emotional state, fever, and medications. Respiratory rhythm refers to the pattern of breathing. This varies with age, with adults being very regular and infants being irregular. The rhythm may be altered by laughing and sighing. Depth of respiration is the amount of air inhaled and exhaled during breathing. It is described as normal, deep, or shallow. It is best observed by watching the rise and fall of the chest wall.

BLOOD PRESSURE

Blood pressure is the pressure of the blood against the walls of the arteries. The measurement consists of two components. The systolic pressure, measured in millimeters of mercury (mm Hg), represents the force exerted on the arterial walls by the blood during the contraction of the ventricles of the heart. It is the higher reading. Diastolic pressure, also measured in millimeters of mercury, represents the force exerted during cardiac relaxation. The average blood pressure of a healthy adult is 120/80 mm Hg, with the generally accepted range of 110/60 mm Hg to 140/90 mm Hg. The numeric difference between the systolic and diastolic reading is known as pulse pressure, which may indicate the tone of the arterial walls. A normal pulse pressure is about 40, with a range of 30 to 50.

As with pulse and respirations, there are many factors that can affect blood pressure. Those that cause an increase in blood pressure include exercise, patient age, pain, smoking, and medications. Decreased blood pressure may be caused by dehydration, sleep, anemia, and gender (women lower than men).

There are two basic pieces of equipment needed to perform a blood pressure. They are a stethoscope and sphygomanometer. The stethoscope

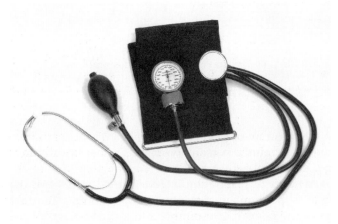

FIGURE 8-3 • Blood pressure equipment.

amplifies the sounds produced by the body and the sphygomanometer measures the pressure of blood in an artery. There are a large variety of sphygomanometers available, some with mercury columns, round dials, and—the newest variety—the acoustic. Figure 8–3 shows a standard blood pressure measurement device.

CLIA '88 WAIVED TESTING

Within the umbrella of the laboratory are several areas where a phlebotomist may gain more skills. These areas include specimen preparation, centrifugation, computer skills (that may include receiving specimens or looking up results), Point-of-Care Testing (POCT), and the Clinical Laboratory Improvements Amendment of 1988 (CLIA '88) waived testing.

CLIA '88 established three categories of laboratory tests based on the complexity of the test. There are personnel standards for each level of testing, but phlebotomists, with further training, are able to perform tests in the category of waived tests. Waived tests, sometimes known as low complexity, are simple to perform, including ones that can be done at home, and require a minimum of judgment and interpretation. (Tests can be moved between categories and revisions are constantly being made.) If a phlebotomist is involved in waived testing procedures, the best way to remain informed is to call the manufacturer of the kits, asking into what category they fall. Also read current literature for any changes. See Chapter 12 for further information concerning CLIA '88. The list found in Table 8–4 is current as of the printing of this book.

POINT-OF-CARE TESTING

Point-of-care testing (POCT) involves the collection and testing of a blood sample, most often a simple capillary puncture, at the site of the patient's care. This type of testing may be done in an operating, emergency or patient room; physician's office; or the patient's own home. The primary purpose of POCT is to decrease turnaround time for blood tests.

The new instruments developed for point-of-care testing are designed to make the tests less dependent on the technical skill of the operator, thus opening the door to the expansion of skills for the phlebotomist. The phlebotomist must be adequately trained, certified, and motivated to do the work. They must also fully appreciate the seriousness of operator error and, therefore, follow strict quality control procedures and be aware of results that may not be correct or of critical value.

Point-of-care testing is constantly evolving. This will involve more phlebotomists, patient care technicians, and others who are willing to learn to operate instruments, perform quality control, and provide accurate results in a timely manner.

GLUCOSE

One of the most common uses of POCT is blood glucose monitoring. Such determination allows the doctor to choose appropriate treatment for patients with diabetes mellitus. Diabetes mellitus is a chronic disease in which the pancreas cannot produce enough insulin or use the insulin that it does produce. Insulin is a chemical released into the bloodstream by the pancreas in response to increased glucose levels in the bloodstream, especially after meals. Insulin allows the glucose from the bloodstream to be absorbed by the tissues, where it is converted into energy. If this process does not—or cannot—occur, the glucose in the bloodstream can

---

TABLE 8-4 • CLIA '88 Waived Tests

- Dipstick urinalysis (nonautomated) for pH, specific gravity, protein, glucose, ketones, blood, bilirubin, urobilogen nitrates, and leukocyte
- Fecal occult blood
- Urine pregnancy testing using visual color comparisons
- Erythrocyte sedimentation rate (nonautomated)
- Hemoglobin (nonautomated)
- Spin hematocrit
- Blood glucose determination with devices approved for home use

---

TABLE 8-5 • Various Point-of-Care Glucose Machines

- Glucometer (Miles Diagnostic Division)
- Accu-Chek (Boehringer Manheim Corp.)
- One Touch (Life Scan)

---

rise to dangerous levels. These high levels can result in strain on major body organs, especially the kidneys; shock; or even death.

Because strict control of glucose levels are necessary in patients with diabetes mellitus, small glucose monitoring machines have become commonplace in the patient's home, doctor's offices, or the hospital bedside. The glucose machines are known by a variety of different names (Table 8–5). These methods require whole blood samples collected by skin puncture from the finger of an adult or the heel of an infant. As with any equipment used to perform testing, adherence to quality control procedures and manufacturer's instructions is of vital importance. Careful recording of results must include date, time, and phlebotomist's initials.

BLOOD GASES AND ELECTROLYTES

Blood gases and electrolytes can also be measured by instruments providing POCT. Blood gas analysis involves measuring the partial pressure of oxygen (PO_2), carbon dioxide (PCO_2), and pH. PO_2 and PCO_2 are measured if a patient has a heart or lung disorder. The blood pH determines if the blood is too acidic or alkaline. These three determinates must be watched closely to determine a patient's respiratory status or monitoring of a patient on oxygen therapy. Along with blood gases, the POCT machinery will often perform blood electrolyte levels such as sodium (Na^+), potassium (K^+), chloride Cl^-), and bicarbonate (HCO_3).

Because the instruments perform more than one test, there are more complex quality control, maintenance, and testing procedures. Also, blood gases are often performed on arterial blood samples so that further training of the phlebotomist may be necessary. (See Chapter 6 for further information.)

COAGULATION

Another test available through POCT is the monitoring of blood coagulation. The most common tests being performed in this manner are prothrombin times (PT) and activated partial thromboplastin times (APTT). Most often, results are obtained through simple capillary puncture and are available within five minutes of testing. Blood coagulation monitoring is of utmost importance in a cardiac catheter laboratory, the operating room, and critical care units. When this type of testing is being performed in an outpatient setting, such as, physician's office or the patient's home visit, it allows for an immediate adjustment of the patient's medication, improves patient compliance, and minimizes laboratory-to-laboratory variability.

HEMOGLOBIN AND HEMATOCRIT

Hemoglobin and hematocrit are tests that have been available as a POCT methodology for quite some time. Most doctors' offices have a hemoglobinometer available to quickly screen for anemia. Also, blood donor centers screen potential donors as to acceptability. Hematocrit centrifuges have long been in use in operating rooms to monitor a patient's blood loss during surgical procedures. Figure 8–4 shows glucose and hemoglobin POCT equipment.

CHOLESTEROL

Cholesterol testing is also available as a POCT instrument. This testing is very often seen as part of a health fair sponsored by a local hospital, clinic, or community college. Given the notoriety about cholesterol, it has been established that there is a direct relationship between high cholesterol levels and heart disease.

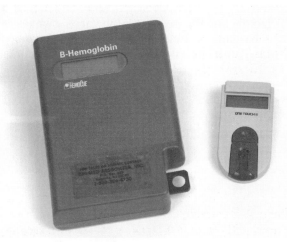

FIGURE 8-4 • Point of care equipment. *(left)* Hemoglobin analysis and *(right)* glucose analysis.

ELECTROCARDIOGRAPHY

Electrocardiography, a graphic recording of the heart's electrical activity, supplies a physician with valuable information about the health of a patient's heart. EKG (or ECG) measures the amount of electrical activity or currents produced by the heart during the process of contraction and relaxation, and the time required for this activity to travel through the heart during each heartbeat.

The following is a brief description as to what is occurring within the heart, what the graphic recording looks like, and what it means. A quick review of the heart's anatomy as found in Chapter 2 is advisable.

To understand an EKG, one must be familiar with the electrical activity of the heart. There are specialized masses of tissue in the heart that form the conduction system. The sinoatrial (SA) node is the body's natural pacemaker. Located in the upper part of the right atrium, it sends out an electrical impulse that begins and regulates the heartbeat.

As each electrical impulse is dispersed, it causes the atria to contract or depolarize. From the atria, the electrical impulse then travels to the atrioventricular (AV) node, then to the bundle of His. This allows the ventricles to fill with blood. The bundle of His divides into right and left branches that allow the electrical impulses to continue traveling to the Purkinje fibers. These fibers evenly distribute the pulse to the right and left ventricles causing them to contract. The heart relaxes briefly, then a new impulse is begun by the SA node, and the cycle starts again. See Figure 8–5.

This cardiac cycle represents one complete heartbeat that consists of a contraction (systole) and relaxation (diastole) of the atria and ventricles. This cycle can be recorded on special paper. The normal EKG cycle consists of waves that have been labeled P, QRS, and T (Fig. 8–6).

The flat horizontal line that separates the various waves is known as the baseline. The baseline is divided into segments for the purpose of interpretation and analysis by the physician. A segment is the portion of

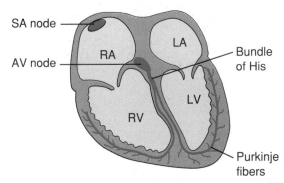

FIGURE 8-5 • Figure depicting the electrical components of the heart.

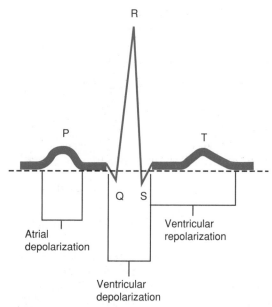

FIGURE 8-6 • Normal EKG cycle highlighting waves.

the EKG between two waves, and an interval is the length of a wave, or the length of a wave with a segment.

The PR interval represents the time it takes from the beginning of the atrial contraction to the beginning of the ventricular contraction. The ST segment represents the time interval from the end of the ventricular depolarization to the beginning of ventricular recovery (repolarization). The QT interval represents the time it takes from the beginning of the ventricular depolarization to the end of the ventricular repolarization. The baseline occurring after a T wave represents the period the heart is resting or in its polarized state. See Figure 8–7.

Each cardiac cycle takes approximately 0.8 seconds for an average of 75 heartbeats per minute. By observing and measuring the size, shape, and location of each wave on an EKG tracing, the doctor can analyze and interpret rate, rhythm, and electrical conduction of the heart. Abnormalities detected in EKG cycles help diagnose cardiac problems such as myocardial infarction (MI), arrhythmias, nodal block, and many other conditions. For further information, a book specifically about EKGs is recommended.

BLOOD DONOR CENTER SKILLS

With a good background in phlebotomy skills, a competent phlebotomist can also be employed in a regional blood center or hospital

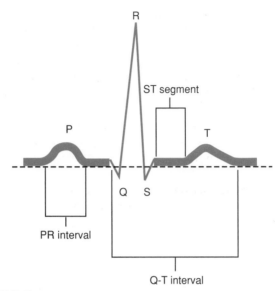

FIGURE 8-7 • Normal EKG cycle highlighting segment and interval.

blood donor center where they screen and collect blood from donors. Work in this type of atmosphere employs many skills, some of which include direct patient contact, interviewing skills, simple physical exam, knowledge of possible donor reactions (such as syncope), aseptic technique, and simple first aid.

Upon arriving, a prospective blood donor will go through a screening process. The phlebotomist will ask questions to first gather demographic information: patient's full name, date of birth (but age only is acceptable), date of last donation (must wait 56 days between donation), and written consent to proceed with the donation process. Following this, a verbal medical history will be taken with questions asked concerning illnesses, whether certain medications have been taken, travel history, recent surgeries, tattoos or body piercing, and sexual history. All these questions will allow the phlebotomist to determine whether the prospective donor is acceptable to give blood, become a temporary deferral for up to three years, or become a permanent deferral.

The next stage is a mini physical exam. This is an area where a multitrained phlebotomist may use many skills. An overall appearance of the donor is noted. A hemoglobin level is checked, usually by the copper sulfate method. Pulse, blood pressure, and temperature are taken. Pulse must be between 50–100 beats per minute. Blood pressure must be no higher than 180/110 mm Hg with pulse pressure between 30–90. Donors with normal blood pressure, but on antihypertensives medication are acceptable. Temperature, taken orally, must not exceed 37.5°C (99.5°F).

As part of the mini-physical, the donor must be weighed. Weight must be at least 110 pounds in order to donate a full unit of blood (450 mL ± 45 mL). This represents 10–13% of the donor's volume.

If a prospective donor passes all of the criteria, he or she may be accepted as a donor. As a final step before actual donation, an informed consent must be signed. The informed consent tells the patient that his or her blood will be tested for infectious diseases such as hepatitis B and antibodies to HIV. The donor would be notified of any positive results and placed on permanent deferral. The donor should understand the entire pre-donation procedure with the opportunity to ask questions and refuse consent.

To perform a venipuncture for the purpose of blood donation, certain procedures must be followed. These are found in Chapter 6.

SUMMARY

No matter what additional skills a phlebotomist may have, the key to obtaining or keeping a job is to be *flexible*. Never rule out any skill, but be willing to crosstrain or take additional courses. Remember, the sky's the limit when it comes to multiskilling.

REVIEW QUESTIONS

1. The four major areas in which a patient's temperature may be taken are: _ORAL_, _RECTAL_, _AXILLARY_, and _AURAL_.

2. Involuntary breathing is controlled by the _MEDULLA OBLONGATA_.

3. The primary purpose of point-of-care testing is _DECREASE TURN AROUND TIME_.

4. A graphic recording of the heart's electrical activity is an _ELECTROCARDIOGRAPHY_.

5. The average pulse rate _DECREASES_ as people mature.

6. _CPR_ is a combination of artificial respiration and circulation.

7. A sphygomanometer and a _STETHOSCOPE_ are needed to ascertain blood pressure.

8. Name three common POCT procedures: _GLUCOSE, BLOOD GASES ELECTROLYTES_, _COAGULATION_, and _CHOLESTEROL_.

PART

II

Professional Issues

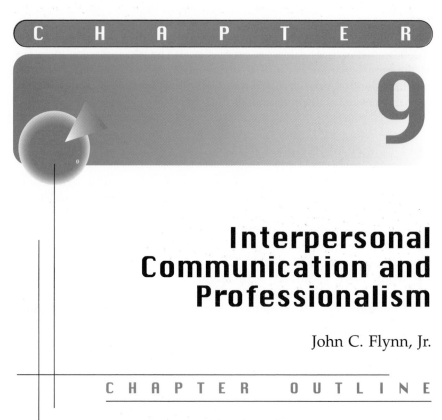

Interpersonal Communication and Professionalism

John C. Flynn, Jr.

The purpose of this chapter is to discuss the importance of interpersonal communication and professionalism in the day-to-day life of a phlebotomist or any health care professional. The two topics are included in the same chapter because they are intricately related. The chapter concludes with a brief discussion of continuing education, a topic that is very important to all professionals.

EFFECTIVE COMMUNICATION

STAT! The word has different meanings for different individuals in the health care setting. To some it means "drop everything and do it now"; to others it means "do it when I can get to it"; and to still others it may mean something else entirely. STAT is a word that is used every day, but in practice the meaning varies from one individual to another and from one department to another. This example of the use (and abuse) of the word STAT illustrates a problem, i.e., effective communication, confronted by phlebotomists.

Communicating is something that laboratory personnel, including phlebotomists, do every day during the course of their jobs. However, the backgrounds of the people with whom they must communicate are very diversified, as illustrated in Chapter 1 (see Fig. 1–3A, B).

In some situations, communication is often thought of as a commodity or substance, as illustrated in the phrase, "we must have more communication"; however, communication is more accurately described as a process, not a commodity. For example, if a plant is lacking water, the situation can be corrected by adding more water. However, if there is a "lack of communication," adding more communication does not necessarily correct the problem; in fact, it can make matters worse. In other words, the trouble with communication problems is not always the *quantity* of communication, but instead the *quality* of the communication.

A LIFE SKILL

There are certain activities common to all people that can be regarded as life skills. These include maintaining one's health and family relationships, self-evaluation and reflection and decision making. Communication is also a life skill, and yet what training do most people receive in communication? Most have had some grade school and secondary school training in English grammar and composition, and perhaps even some speech training, but generally no interpersonal communications training, which is what phlebotomists, and all laboratory workers, must use daily.

Laboratory and health care workers must realize that there are several levels of communication, all of which must be used properly to do their job well. First is what may be called *intrapersonal* communication. This is the ability to see ourselves as others see us—in other words, "being in someone else's shoes." It also includes the ability to think and plan in advance how to react in a given situation. Second, there is *one-way* communication. An example of this is the sometimes annoying memos or notes received from supervisors, **subordinates,** or peers. These, if not written properly, are open to improper interpretation. Finally, there is *interpersonal* (two-way) communication, which is the level at which phlebotomists and laboratorians communicate most frequently.

KEYS TO SUCCESSFUL COMMUNICATION

Before interpersonal communication can be successful, there are certain fundamental conditions that must be present. First, both parties must be attentive and willing to engage in the communication process. Did you ever try to talk about something to a friend, supervisor, patient or coworker and at some point notice that they tuned you out? Or rather than listening to you, they are constantly looking at their watch or a clock or gazing out a window? These experiences can be very frustrating and counter productive. Therefore, in addition to being a good communicator, the importance of being a good listener cannot be overlooked.

Second, both parties must act as senders and receivers of messages. Once an individual receives a message (by being a good listener) he or she must then become a sender and let the other party know that the message was received and understood, or that more information is needed. This is very important. If a message is received and not clearly understood, it is imperative that clarification or further instruction be requested. The two participants are interdependent; for the communication process to be complete, they must interact.

Finally, and most importantly in the health care setting, communication must be based on mutual understanding. This implies that a given phrase or term, such as "type and hold," means the same thing to both parties. We all have had the experience of being misunderstood because the person we were talking with interpreted something differently from the way we intended. Laboratory personnel must be careful when using **jargon,** which, although used daily in the laboratory, may not be understood outside the laboratory setting.

OBSTACLES TO SUCCESSFUL COMMUNICATION

Unfortunately, all people encounter barriers to effective communication. One of these is distrust. Distrust can lead to defensive interpersonal communication, especially when the recipient perceives the communication as an attempt to control, manipulate or when a problem is being addressed. Additionally, if the sender has a superior attitude, this will trigger a defensive response. Distrust can be overcome if questions or directives are communicated in a nonthreatening way that makes the issue a mutual problem. In this manner, respect and equality are communicated to recipients, giving them the feeling that their help and judgment are valued.

Another common barrier that hinders effective communication is a reference gap. This is analogous to a generation gap or racial gap, in which background and environments affect the way people think, perceive the world or environment, and, in this case, communicate. Phlebotomists have a different frame of reference from others with whom they must communicate, including laboratory personnel in other departments, nurses, physicians, social workers, and patients. For example, you may wonder why a test is ordered STAT. Your frame of reference is different from that of the physician; the physician obviously knows something about the patient that you do not know. Similarly, when you are asked by a physician why a STAT request is not done, you may have to explain that all tests from their service were ordered STAT (an abuse of the STAT designation) or that an emergency has arisen, thereby communicating to them your frame of reference.

Oftentimes, participants of health care teams take part in group discussions or decision making. Disagreement with an idea that you have put forth should not be interpreted as personal dislike. This is unhealthy, another barrier to effective communication, and it must be realized that everyone involved in the process have the best intentions, whether the decision is regarding a patient or where to put a new piece of equipment. Furthermore, it should be remembered that in a group process, generally the ultimate decision is usually the best one.

One final issue to be addressed is the use, or often the misuse, of body language. After the spoken word, our eyes are the most potent communicator we possess. For example, rolling eyes say one thing, and tear-filled eyes, another; surprise, disappointment, and anger are all expressions and feelings we can communicate with our eyes. Reluctance to make eye contact also sends a message to the recipient. Therefore, communication must be both verbal and nonverbal. This is especially important for a phlebotomist, who must interact with patients.

Therefore, be sure to make eye contact when speaking or listening to patients. Avoid constant monitoring of the time by either looking at your wristwatch or checking a wall clock. Avoid deep sighs or fidgeting with a pencil, sorting supplies, reading or tapping your toe, all of which signal boredom or impatience. Avoid assuming a defensive posture such as crossing your arms. Your aim is to put the patient at ease, which is best accomplished by acting confident, maintaining eye contact when speaking or listening to a patient or colleague, and appearing relaxed.

COMMUNICATION BREAKDOWN

In most instances, communication between the phlebotomist and others goes rather smoothly. Communication works well, for example, when a physician or nurse calls for testing results, to determine whether blood is ready for the next day's operation schedule, or to inquire about what color tube is needed for a given test. In these generally relaxed situations, communication is open and friendly. Communication breaks down during times of increased stress, the very times when it is most critical that communication be very smooth. A classic example is when an emergency is occurring either in the emergency department or in the operating room and there is a strain in the communication chain between these places and the laboratory. Someone may ask for results of a test that was never ordered or question why blood is not ready for a trauma victim when the phlebotomist was never informed that there was a trauma patient or that he or she needed to collect a specimen. However, with patience and self-control, the communication process will work even during times of stress.

GENERAL GUIDELINES FOR EFFECTIVE COMMUNICATION

First, communication should be open and honest. This applies whether you are a subordinate or a supervisor, and the key is respect and courtesy for the individual with whom you are communicating. Glibness, deceptiveness, sarcasm, etc., have no place during communication if you wish to be taken seriously.

Second, avoid generalizations and **stereotyping.** We have all been guilty of this at some time, whether it was regarding someone in the health care field or of another race or ethnic group. Talk to the *individual,* for that is what he or she deserves.

Third, consider your "environment" or frame of reference. Explain where you are "coming from," including the pressures and time constraints you are under. It is equally important to consider the environment of the individual with whom you are communicating.

Finally, communicate with a humanistic approach. In addition to the above guidelines, one should be sensitive or sympathetic to other concerns or problems. Oftentimes, all a frustrated patient or coworker desires is to have someone listen to them.

TABLE 9-1 • General Guidelines for Effective Communication
1. Be open and honest. 2. Avoid generalizations. 3. Consider environments. 4. Use a humanistic approach. 5. Be a good listener.

These guidelines, which are the hallmarks of professional behavior, are summarized in Table 9–1.

In some situations these guidelines cannot be observed. We may be under pressure or short of time, but we must keep in mind that we are dealing with another individual who may not be aware of our circumstances or situation. When the circumstances improve, it is recommended to contact the person with whom we may have been "short" or impatient, explain the situation that led to our abruptness, and thank the person for his or her cooperation and patience. This way we are not forgetting our obligation to a fellow health care provider to be courteous, professional, and, above all else, human.

PROFESSIONALISM

Historically, there were three professions—the law, medicine, and theology (the three "robed" professions)—and three types of professions—lawyers, doctors, and clergymen. In the nineteenth and twentieth centuries, the field of professionals greatly expanded to include businesspeople, accountants, computer programmers, social workers, and people in all areas of health care, to name a few.

Strictly speaking, a profession is an area or field that has (1) a distinct field of knowledge requiring specialized training or education; (2) a full-time occupation, often defined and regulated by a peer organization; (3) an occupation that has a service orientation; and (4) a high degree of autonomy. Today, an increasing number of occupations call themselves professions. Phlebotomy became a profession when it moved from being a task or procedure of clinical laboratory personnel (MT/CLS and MLT/CLT) to being performed by specialists, those referred to today as phlebotomists.

Regardless of the definition of a profession, anyone can act professionally while conducting business or employment duties. Professionalism can be thought of as a state of mind. In this sense, acting as a professional encompasses how you look, act, communicate, and present yourself. For a phlebotomist, being well dressed and well groomed is one key to looking like a professional; but looking good is only part of the picture. How you communicate with superiors, peers, and patients and their families is obviously very important to acting professionally. How you conduct yourself and handle adversity will further define whether you act professionally. Obviously, if you throw fits or temper tantrums, act defensively, etc., you are not acting professionally.

One aspect of most professions is the incorporation of a creed or code of ethics into their training. For example, physicians have the Hippocratic oath. However, this oath or creed does not have to be a formal one, but it should include a set of standards to abide by. As discussed in Chapter 1, the American Society for Clinical Laboratory Science (ASCLS) has published a code of ethics that can also be applied to phlebotomists; in summary, this code states that confidentiality will be maintained; duties will be carried out with "accuracy, thoughtfulness and care"; and conduct will always be of a high standard.

Ethical or professional conduct, in general, also includes respect for patients and their rights as outlined in the *Patient's Bill of Rights* (Table 9–2); refraining from discussing patients outside of the proper environment; refraining from anything other than professional communication with patients; and a willingness to assist others.

Finally, one characteristic of a profession is the certification or credentialing of its members. Certification indicates that the individual has mastered the body of knowledge associated with the given profession. Additionally, it gives employers some assurance that a potential employee has baseline skills and can more quickly become a productive member of the health care team. Table 9–3 lists the various organizations that offer certification examinations for phlebotomists.

CONTINUING EDUCATION

Once phlebotomists are credentialed and certified, they should not "rest on their laurels." As defined earlier, a profession includes a distinct field of knowledge. Knowledge is not stagnant, and what is regarded as today's truth may be tomorrow's fiction. New theories and methods are being discovered and tested every day on topics ranging from losing weight, to treating patients and illness, and to coping with stress. This is also true in phlebotomy; some examples of changes include the use of evacuated tubes instead of syringes, and keeping the arm straight rather than bent after collecting a blood specimen.

Once you are credentialed and working, how do you learn about new techniques and changes in the field? Some learn from sale representatives, by attending workshops, or by having inservice programs at their place of employment. This type of learning is known as continuing education (CE).

TABLE 9-2 • Patient's Bill of Rights*

1. The patient has the right to considerate and respectful care.
2. The patient has the right to and is encouraged to obtain from physicians and other direct caregivers relevant, current, and understandable information concerning diagnosis, treatment, and prognosis.

    Except in emergencies when the patient lacks decision-making capacity and the need for treatment is urgent, the patient is entitled to the opportunity to discuss and request information related to the specific procedures and/or treatments, the risks involved, the possible length of recuperation, and the medically reasonable alternatives and their accompanying risks and benefits.

    Patients have the right to know the identity of physicians, nurses, and others involved in their care, as well as when those involved are students, residents, or other trainees. The patient also has the right to know the immediate and long-term financial implications of treatment choices, insofar as they are known.
3. The patient has the right to make decisions about the plan of care prior to and during the course of treatment and to refuse a recommended treatment or plan of care to the extent permitted by law and hospital policy and to be informed of the medical consequences of this action. In case of such refusal, the patient is entitled to other appropriate care and services that the hospital provides or transfer to another hospital. The hospital should notify patients of any policy that might affect patient choice within the institution.
4. The patient has the right to have an advance directive (such as a living will, health care proxy, or durable power of attorney for health care) concerning treatment or designating a surrogate decision maker with the expectation that the hospital will honor the intent of that directive to the extent permitted by law and hospital policy.

    Health care institutions must advise patients of their rights under state law and hospital policy to make informed medical choices, ask if the patient has an advance directive, and include that information in patient records. The patient has the right to timely information about hospital policy that may limit its ability to implement fully a legally valid advance directive.
5. The patient has the right to every consideration of privacy. Case discussion, consultation, examination, and treatment should be conducted so as to protect each patient's privacy.
6. The patient has the right to expect that all communications and records pertaining to his/her care will be treated as confidential by the hospital, except in cases such as suspected abuse and public health hazards when reporting is permitted or required by law. The patient has the right to expect that the hospital will emphasize the confidentiality of this information when it releases it to any other parties entitled to review information in these records.

TABLE 9-2 • Patient's Bill of Rights* (Continued)

7. The patient has the right to review the records pertaining to his/her medical care and to have the information explained or interpreted as necessary, except when restricted by law.
8. The patient has the right to expect that, within its capacity and policies, a hospital will make reasonable response to the request of a patient for appropriate and medically indicated care and services. The hospital must provide evaluation, service, and/or referral as indicated by the urgency of the case. When medically appropriate and legally permissible, or when a patient has so requested, a patient may be transferred to another facility. The institution to which the patient is to be transferred must first have accepted the patient for transfer. The patient must also have the benefit of complete information and explanation concerning the need for, risks, benefits, and alternatives to such a transfer.
9. The patient has the right to ask and be informed of the existence of business relationships among the hospital, educational institutions, other health care providers, or payers that may influence the patient's treatment and care.
10. The patient has the right to consent to or decline to participate in proposed research studies or human experimentation affecting care and treatment or requiring direct patient involvement, and to have those studies fully explained prior to consent. A patient who declines to participate in research or experimentation is entitled to the most effective care that the hospital can otherwise provide.
11. The patient has the right to expect reasonable continuity of care when appropriate and to be informed by physicians and other caregivers of available and realistic patient care options when hospital care is no longer appropriate.
12. The patient has the right to be informed of hospital policies and practices that relate to patient care, treatment, and responsibilities. The patient has the right to be informed of available resources for resolving disputes, grievances, and conflicts, such as ethics committees, patient representatives, or other mechanisms available in the institution. The patient has the right to be informed of the hospital's charges for services and available payment methods.

The collaborative nature of health care requires that patients, or their families/surrogates, participate in their care. The effectiveness of care and patient satisfaction with the course of treatment depend, in part, on the patient fulfilling certain responsibilities. Patients are responsible for providing information about past illnesses, hospitalizations, medications, and other matters related to health status. To participate effectively in decision making, patients must be encouraged to take responsibility for requesting additional information or clarification about their health status or treatment when they do not fully understand information and instructions. Patients

Table continued on following page

TABLE 9-2 • **Patient's Bill of Rights*** *(Continued)*

are also responsible for ensuring that the health care institution has a copy of their written advance directive if they have one. Patients are responsible for informing their physicians and other caregivers if they anticipate problems in following prescribed treatment.

Patients should also be aware of the hospital's obligation to be reasonably efficient and equitable in providing care to other patients and the community. The hospital's rules and regulations are designed to help the hospital meet this obligation. Patients and their families are responsible for making reasonable accommodations to the needs of the hospital, other patients, medical staff, and hospital employees. Patients are responsible for providing necessary information for insurance claims and for working with the hospital to make payment arrangements, when necessary.

A person's health depends on much more than health care services. Patients are responsible for recognizing the impact of their life-style on their personal health.

Conclusion

Hospitals have many functions to perform, including the enhancement of health status, health promotion, and the prevention and treatment of injury and disease; the immediate and ongoing care and rehabilitation of patients; the education of health professionals, patients, and the community; and research. All these activities must be conducted with an overriding concern for the values and dignity of patients.

Reprinted with permission of the American Hospital Association, copyright 1992.
*These rights can be exercised on the patient's behalf by a designated surrogate or proxy decision maker if the patient lacks decision-making capacity, is legally incompetent, or is a minor.

CE is rapidly growing in importance. Physicians, lawyers, teachers and those in many other professional groups participate in CE and are often required to accumulate CE credits. (Generally, it takes 8 to 10 hours of contact time, depending on the organization, to earn one continuing education unit [CEU].) Once you are certified, some organizations, such as the American Society for Clinical Laboratory Science and the American Society of Phlebotomy Technicians, require accumulation of CEUs to maintain certification. Many other certification and credentialing organizations do not require CE, but they all strongly encourage it. Additionally, the Joint Commission on Accreditation of Healthcare Organizations (JCAHO) requires inservice training.

Most of the above-mentioned organizations provide educational experiences for individuals to earn CEUs, such as workshops at local and national meetings, videoconferences, audioconferences, and self-instructional units. Other noncredentialing organizations, such as the

American Association of Blood Banks and the American Association of Clinical Chemistry, offer CE that is recognized by the credentialing organizations. Still other organizations, such as the National Laboratory Training Network, American Society of Clinical Pathologists, and the Area Health Education Center, provide educational opportunities for laboratory personnel. The Mayo Medical Laboratories also offer workshops for phlebotomists at various locations around the country.

As you can see, there is ample opportunity for phlebotomists to acquire CE. As a professional, you should want to continue your education and keep abreast of changes and new technologies in your field. In addition, not only should you attend your organization's CE offerings, but you should also become active in your organization. Volunteer to assist at workshops by organizing and scheduling speakers, rooms, or refreshments. Do not "rest on your laurels." Instead, attend CE (you may not have a choice), and become active in the organization of your choice.

Finally, as discussed in Chapter 8, multiskilling and cross-training are the current trends. Some feel that phlebotomy-only technicians will soon be a thing of the past. While this may be a trend, there will always be a need for the well-trained, proficient phlebotomist.

TABLE 9-3 • Phlebotomy Certification Examination Options

American Society of Clinical Pathologists (ASCP)
2100 West Harrison Street
Chicago, IL 60612-3798
(This is probably the most popular examination.)

National Credentialing Agency for Laboratory Personnel (NCA)
P.O. Box 15945-289
Lenexa, KS 66285-5945
(Offered in cooperation with the ASCLS)

American Society of Phlebotomy Technicians (ASPT)
P.O. Box 1831
Hickory, NC 28603

National Phlebotomy Association (NPA)
2623 Bladenburg Road NE
Washington, DC 20018

National Healthcareer Association
194 Route 46E
Fairfield, NJ 07004

REVIEW QUESTIONS

1. Activities such as maintaining one's health, self-evaluation, and decision making are examples of ___LIFE SKILLS___ .

2. The ability to see ourselves as others see us is known as ___INTRAPERSONAL___ communication.

3. When our background and environment are different from those who we communicate with, this can be referred to as a ___REFERENCE GAP___ .

4. An occupation with a high degree of autonomy, service orientation, and specialized training is known as a ___PROFESSION___ .

5. ___CONTINUING EDUCATION___ is an activity that is provided by most employers and professional organizations.

Bibliography

Barrack MK: How We Communicate; The Most Vital Skill. Macomb, IL, Glenbridge Publishing, 1988.

Duldt BW, Giffin K, Patton BR: Interpersonal Communication in Nursing. Philadelphia, FA Davis, 1984.

Ellis A, Beattie G: The Psychology of Language and Communication. New York, Guilford Press, 1986.

Ernst DJ: Is the phlebotomist obsolete? *MLO* 29(10):30–34, 1997.

Gazda GM, Childers WC, Walters RP: Interpersonal Communication: A Handbook for Health Professionals. Rockville, MD, Aspen, 1982.

Giffin K, Patton BR: Fundamentals of Interpersonal Communication. 2nd ed. New York, Harper & Row, 1976.

Walton D: Are You Communicating? You Can't Manage Without It. New York, McGraw-Hill, 1989.

Weaver RL: Understanding Interpersonal Communication. 2nd ed. Glenview, IL, Scott, Foresman, 1978.

Phlebotomy Department Management

Dorothy Pfender

- **Maintaining Quality**
  Record Keeping
  Continuing Education
  Communication
  Employee Performance and Review

- **Budgeting**

- **Summary**

The phlebotomy department is the foundation of the clinical laboratory. Laboratory test results are valuable only if the specimens are from the correct patient, properly collected, labeled, handled, and transported. The department acts as a liaison between the laboratory and hospital departments, physicians, patients, and the public. In fact, public opinion of the laboratory is often based on the treatment received from the phlebotomy department.

The manager of this department should possess all the standard managerial training and skills. They should have special expertise in relating to people: communicating, listening, and adapting. Organizational skill is critical since they must correlate the work of the department with the functions of nurses, doctors, therapists, etc., and the technical units of the laboratory while considering the patients' comforts. In addition, they must have training and skill in the techniques used in the department and some understanding of the performance and meaning of the tests performed in the laboratory. Budgeting and financial expertise is extremely important in these days of changing medical care payment systems.

ORGANIZATION

PLANNING

When planning a phlebotomy department, the following should be considered:

1. Number of patients to be served
2. Source of patients (e.g., hospital, physicians' offices, health promotion programs, mass screening, employee physicals)

3. Type of patient (e.g., age, ethnic and religious background, economic status, and whether the patient is in the hospital or ambulatory)

4. Location of the laboratory or laboratories to which specimens will be sent

5. Type of specimens the department will be collecting (blood, urine, cultures from various sources, blood requiring special pre- or post-treatment, or other bodily excrements)

6. The responsibility associated with transporting specimens

7. Availability and type of computer system and how involved the department will be in its use, i.e., who will be responsible for originating patient data and/or keeping it current? Will there be preprinted labels and/or instructions with the requisitions, etc.?

8. The responsibility and involvement with screening tests

9. How involved will the phlebotomy department be in "off site" collecting

10. If "Point-of-Care Units" exist, what will be the responsibilities of the phlebotomist

11. Where stock supplies are stored

The information necessary for these considerations can be obtained from the following sources:

1. Hospital administrators

2. Hospital statistics

3. Local or hospital-based physicians

4. Nurses

5. Laboratory directors, managers, and statistics

6. Other skilled health departments (e.g., radiology, respiratory medicine, physical therapy, and nutrition)

LOCATION AND FACILITIES

The location and physical layout of the phlebotomy unit are important. The unit should be easily accessible to **ambulatory** patients from the central registration area and the outside entrance. It should also be located so that phlebotomists have easy access to the emergency department and elevators to patient areas.

The phlebotomy unit should have a reception area that is readily visible to people entering the unit. Requests of ambulatory patients are reviewed here and all necessary patient information obtained and recorded. A computer system (the hospital's or the unit's) is recommended for this work. Ambulatory traffic through the unit is directed from this area. All telephone calls are received here and directed to the proper location.

There should be a paging system or "beepers" available for use by phlebotomists when they are out of the unit area. It is a good idea to have a system by which phlebotomists keep the control desk aware of their location so that they can be informed of new requests received from that area or from an area they will pass on their way back to the laboratory. This increases efficiency and prevents irritation.

Ideally, there should be a phlebotomy information and work organization center. Here requests can be sorted, work organized, and collection notes made. In addition, special instructions and communications can be posted here.

The actual venipuncture area should be private and should contain a comfortable chair for the patient with an area on which to place either arm comfortably. The armrest areas should be at a comfortable height for the phlebotomist; most phlebotomy chairs have adjustable arms. Each area should be equipped with a "panic button" or some other system of requesting help if needed. Ammonia inhalants and, if possible, oxygen should be available. There should be adequate supplies neatly stored, as well as a sink and biohazard disposal containers in each area. It is advantageous to provide an examination table or a way of allowing the patient to lie down if required. A place should be provided in each area to hang patients' coats; a couple of hooks and a few hangers are usually sufficient. If patients must hang their coats outside the venipuncture area, a secure place should be provided nearby to put patients more at ease.

The ideal phlebotomy area will have a place where the patient can lie down, if needed, such as a cot, bed, or reclining phlebotomy chair. When each venipuncture area cannot be equipped with a place for the patient to lie down, there must be at least one such area centrally located (1) for patients undergoing a blood test that requires rest before the specimen is collected and (2) for those who experience adverse reactions. Oxygen and ammonia inhalants should be readily available in the central reclining area. Ideally, all venipuncture areas should be soundproof. This allows private discussions and reactions to the procedures. If children or mentally retarded patients are treated, at least one soundproof room should be available.

Restrooms should be adequate and should be located next to or across the hall from the venipuncture areas. Each restroom should be equipped with some type of emergency call system. Convenient shelf space should be provided for containers and other equipment used before and after collecting the specimen.

It is often advantageous to have the patient collect a urine specimen while waiting for the phlebotomist. The container to be used should be labeled when it is given to the patient. To prevent embarrassment, provide a place where the patient may leave the labeled specimen before returning to the waiting room. This should be convenient to the restrooms and venipuncture areas.

STAFFING

WORKLOAD UNITS

The staffing pattern will differ for each phlebotomy unit. The College of American Pathologists (CAP) and other organizations have published rules for determining how many employee hours are needed and have determined weighted time units called workload units for each test. One unit represents "one minute of technical, clinical, and aide time" needed for a procedure (Table 10–1). These published figures can only be used as guidelines. Because there are so many variables, each unit must evaluate its own situation and determine its own workload units and needs.

To make this determination, the following factors should be considered:

1. Volume of specimens. This is not the number of patients, but the number of tests ordered on each patient. For example, it will take less time to collect blood for a blood glucose test on each of 10 patients than to collect blood for a blood glucose test and a complete blood cell (CBC) count on each of 10 patients.

2. Number and location of patients.

3. Type of patients (i.e., ambulatory patients or inpatients). For inpatients, the time required to reach their room or to go from room to room must be considered. The place of collection (i.e., regular hospital room or special areas) must also be considered. Isolation units or intensive care units, for example, require

TABLE 10–1 • Sample of Cap Workload Units

Procedure	Workload Units
Capillary puncture on outpatient	8.0
Capillary puncture on inpatient	14.0
Venipuncture on outpatient	4.0
Venipuncture on inpatient	10.0

special preparations to work in them. Even in regular rooms, the problems that the phlebotomist encounters in accessing the patient because of the arrangement of furniture, equipment in use, and the presence of visitors should be considered. Children, elderly patients, and burned or trauma patients may also require more time.

4. Method of labeling specimens (preprinted labels or hand written).

5. The amount of work that can be done at scheduled collection times.

6. The number of STAT or special collections that are required.

7. The size of the emergency department, trauma unit, and other specific patient units. In some hospitals, one or all of these units may be large enough to support an assigned phlebotomist or person to handle the transportation of specimens.

8. Whether the department offers 24-hour coverage or has another department cover evening and night hours.

9. Duties other than collecting specimens (i.e., transporting, logging-in, centrifuging specimens, and preparing specimens to be picked up or mailed).

10. What screening tests will the phlebotomy department be responsible for, where they are done, how they are reported, etc.? Who is responsible for maintaining the equipment used for them and the quality control?

11. How involved will the phlebotomy department be with "Point-of-Care" units.

Experience has proven that it is most efficient to have a core of full-time employees to cover the basic needs and a staff of part-time employees for peak hours and other times of staff shortages. The manager should try to schedule enough phlebotomists so that they do not feel constantly pushed, but not so many that they are bored. Be realistic when allotting time required to collect specimens.

TRAINING AND PROFESSIONAL ATTRIBUTES

Employ formally trained phlebotomists if possible, and develop an orientation and instruction program for these employees; generally 2 weeks are sufficient. This program should be longer, if necessary, to familiarize the employee with the methods, procedures, and general operating protocol of the department. A department manual should be provided, and employees should understand that uniformity is necessary. Physicians compare results of tests done before and after treatment, and uniformity of test performance is necessary for these comparisons to be valid. If you employ less experienced phlebotomists, the orientation and training period must be longer and more in depth.

In addition to formal education and training, phlebotomists should possess the following professional attributes:

1. Professional appearance
2. Ability to relate well to people by showing concern and being courteous
3. Professional attitude
4. Ability to remain calm during emergencies
5. Capacity to accept changes
6. Willingness to adhere to the rules of the department
7. Understands the need to admit to any errors and take steps to correct them

OPERATIONAL PLAN

It is important to develop goals and objectives for the department. The hospital or clinic will probably have general goals with which you will be expected to identify. However, more specific goals are needed to develop an efficient, successful department. The primary goal of every phlebotomy department is to contribute to good patient care by obtaining proper (good) specimens for the test requested by the physician. This means that specimens must be collected from the proper patient, at the correct time, using the proper technique; all specimens must be labeled correctly and transported in a timely manner to the testing department. A well-organized system of handling requests, specimen collection, and carefully established techniques is required to accomplish this goal.

The phlebotomy department shares servicing the patient with radiology, respiratory therapy, physical therapy, nursing, physicians, and possibly others. A good operational plan requires consideration of the functions and routines of these departments.

Occasionally, reorganization of a well-functioning operational plan will be necessary to accommodate changes in the hospital, laboratory, and/or the phlebotomy department. Have all departments review the proposed changes for possible conflicts. If any conflicts arise, resolve them before instituting the change. Provide all departments with the necessary facts of the change and when it will become effective, and distribute this information in writing.

It is important that all staff members feel they are part of a team and work as such. This necessitates that each department understand and respect the work requirements of the others. Regular meetings with managers or representatives from all departments are recommended. The requirements of the procedures in each department should be discussed. When there are conflicts, reasons why changes can or cannot be made should be presented. Departments must work together to reach solutions that allow each department to organize its work satisfactorily. Usually, the phlebotomy department must take the initiative in this team effort, as it is the department most affected by the work of all other departments. If you are honest about your needs and try to be flexible, others will usually follow this example, and a mutually satisfactory work organization can be developed.

Explain to the employees the reasons for any compromises either by your department or by others. This will develop a good rapport among all departments. This approach helps to create an understanding and respect for the employees and needs of all departments, yours included.

HANDLING REQUESTS

The process of handling requests is dependent on the system used to create and receive them. The handling procedure in your department should be such that the requests are promptly sorted and allocated so as to assure timely and proper attention.

COLLECTION SCHEDULE

A specified time for early morning specimen collection (i.e., morning rounds) is a given in all hospitals. At this time routine, fasting, and presurgical specimens are collected. The time of collection and the number of employees involved varies, depending on the following:

1. When the laboratory wants the specimen. If the laboratory day shift starts at 7 A.M. and these technicians set up the instruments, they will not be ready for the specimens until sometime after 7 A.M. If the night technicians set up the instruments and the day shift starts at 7 A.M., the laboratory will be ready for specimens at 7 A.M.

2. Who is responsible for recording and preparing specimens for analysis. If a department other than the analyzing department

does this, it will need the specimens at a time that will allow it to meet the laboratory starting time.

3. Volume of specimens, including the number (how many tubes) and type (do they require special handling?).

4. Number and location of patients. Are they in rooms that are close to each other? Are they in special areas that require special preparation?

5. Type of patient (e.g., children, elderly patients, or burn patients).

6. When breakfast is served.

The morning collection usually starts between 5:30 and 7:00 A.M. Several other collection times scheduled throughout the day will help with the organization of the work. Three other scheduled collection times are recommended: mid-morning, mid-afternoon, and early evening. The times chosen for scheduled rounds will be determined by the routines of the other departments involved in the patient's care and the laboratory performing the test. The schedule set up should be strictly adhered to and known by all departments involved. Many phone calls and false STATS will be eliminated when there is a dependable, known schedule. A frequently used schedule is a collection at 11:00 A.M., 2:30 P.M., and 7:00 P.M. All requests received in the laboratory up to 15 minutes before a scheduled collection will be included in that collection.

STAT and other special collection requests are a big part of every day's work. It is impossible to predict how many and when these requests will be received. It seems logical to have them handled by whoever is not busy at the time the requests are received. This works well unless everyone or no one is busy. When no one is busy, some people never volunteer, causing friction in the staff. When everyone is busy, there is time lost deciding who can best interrupt what they are doing. A satisfactory system for responding to STATS will be unique to each department. Basically, the person or persons who should respond to STATS must be decided before, *not* after, the STAT request is received. The phlebotomists should know the schedule and it should be posted so there is no indecision about who is responsible. Make the STAT assignments as equitable as possible. Honor requests for assignments, and check regularly to be sure that assignments are satisfactory to the entire staff and you. A system that has worked well is to assign a phlebotomist as primary responder and one as backup for 2-hour periods. Repeat the assignments throughout the day, if necessary, but separate them by at least 2 hours. The "STAT phlebotomist" can be involved with interruptable work of the department.

Special and timed collections can be integrated in the routine collections when possible. Otherwise, someone should be responsible for making sure they are handled correctly.

ESTABLISHING TECHNIQUES

When establishing techniques for tests, it is best to obtain input from the persons and departments using the tests. The ideal technique will meet both your and their needs. Let them review your decision. When a technique has been established, it should be followed. In some instances (e.g., Ivy bleeding time tests), uniformity is essential for the results to be useful to the physician. Minor variations that do not affect test results may be acceptable. Variations should be kept at a minimum. The more uniform the department's techniques, the better its performance can be evaluated.

EQUIPMENT MANAGEMENT

The equipment, both expendable and **capital,** used in the phlebotomy department should be chosen carefully. The decision regarding what to obtain should be made in cooperation with the phlebotomists and in line with budget considerations. All equipment should be monitored and records kept so it can be evaluated and changes made if indicated.

EXPENDABLE EQUIPMENT

Expendables should be chosen carefully after the unit manager and the phlebotomists have used them and discussed their advantages and disadvantages. Do not buy based on price alone, and choose only one kind. Uniformity of equipment is economical, space saving, and important to the operation of the department. Stock the variety of sizes that you need from the same manufacturer whenever possible. See Table 10–2 for a list of expendables.

Storage space is almost always a problem. All products are dated, and you should have approximately 2 months' supply on hand. Determine from statistics and operating experience what your yearly need will be. When you place an order for a year's supply, you are assured that the product will be there for you. Generally, you will also receive bulk and guaranteed pricing for the year. Make an agreement with your supplier to deliver your order in designated portions at designated intervals. A good plan is to have one-thirteenth of your yearly order delivered at a given

TABLE 10-2 • Examples of Expendable Equipment

Needles	Adhesive bandages
Syringes	Glass slides
Lancets	Gloves
Tubes	Biohazard/sharps containers
Tourniquets	Labeling pens
Alcohol, alcohol pads	Special labels/precautions
Povidone-iodine swabs	Puncture site warmers
Cotton balls	Ammonia inhalants
Gauze, sterile pads	Clay sealer
Adhesive tape	

date, another delivery 2 weeks later, and remaining deliveries every 4 weeks afterward.

Expendable supplies used in small quantities should be ordered at intervals, with quantities determined by usage, storage space, and order processing and delivery time. It is wise to keep at least 2 weeks' supply in stock.

CAPITAL EQUIPMENT

Collection trays are a vital piece of capital equipment; each phlebotomist should have his or her own. The organizing and stocking of the tray is very personal, and phlebotomists prefer not to share trays. The collection volume and the space in which they are used and stored must be considered when selecting size and shape. The construction and weight of the tray is also an important consideration.

Capital equipment should be evaluated carefully before purchasing and while in use. Consider the following:

1. How well it meets your needs
2. Accuracy
3. Reproducibility
4. Ease of operation
5. Ease of maintenance
6. Available service
7. Whether quality control is available

It is important to see the equipment demonstrated and, when possible, to obtain opinions from other users. See Table 10–3 for a list of capital equipment that may be needed for a phlebotomy unit.

TABLE 10-3 • Examples of Capital Equipment

Collection trays
Venipuncture chairs
Beds or other reclining surfaces
Utility carts and cabinets
Refrigerators
File cabinets
Computer
Blood pressure cuffs
Racks for tubes
Glucose screening instruments
Hemogloubin and/or hematocrit screening instruments
Beepers and/or communication system
Alarm systems
Timers
Stopwatches
Centrifuges

INVENTORY

Maintain an inventory of all supplies and equipment. A biweekly inventory of expendables will serve to alert you to unexpected shortages and excesses. This allows time to order or change prescheduled deliveries. Capital equipment should be labeled and records kept of its location, use, and maintenance. A yearly inventory of capital equipment is recommended.

MAINTAINING QUALITY

Safety, quality control, and quality assurance programs should be developed to maintain quality. If the phlebotomy department is responsible for the instruments used for screening tests, it should be arranged to have the laboratory run duplicate tests periodically in addition to the manufacturer's recommended quality control. Knowledge of the correlation of the tests performed by the laboratory and the screening tests is useful to the physician when both are used to determine proper dosage. Guidelines for these programs are supplied by the Joint Commission on Accreditation of Healthcare Organizations (JCAHO), the College of American Pathologists (CAP), and the Occupational Safety and Health Administration (OSHA).

All infection control and safety rules of the hospital are applicable to the phlebotomy department and should be enforced.

RECORD KEEPING

Records should be kept of:

- Work performed
- Schedules
- Incidents
- Preventive maintenance
- Equipment repair
- Purchasing information
- Quality controls

JCAHO, CAP, and OSHA provide you with information necessary to establish acceptable necessary records. Accrediting agencies and the federal government have established mandatory periods of time for which all records must be kept available. This varies, but 5 years is the most common requirement.

Practical and useful systems for monitoring the safety, quality control, and quality assurance programs of the department should be established. Such monitoring can point out weak areas in planning, organizing, budgeting, etc., as well as the progress and successes of the department. The value of these records should be explained to the staff. Review these records regularly, and share your opinion of their meaning with the members of the department. Be sure to commend staff members when results are good, and thoroughly discuss any indicated improvement when results are less than acceptable.

CONTINUING EDUCATION

As discussed in Chapter 9, a system of continuing education should also be developed and implemented. Make available to employees information about advances in the areas of health care in which they are involved. Encourage them also to become familiar with developments in other areas of health care. Encourage attendance at seminars and workshops by providing financial aid and an equitable distribution of opportunity. Be sure you, as a manager, attend seminars and workshops and keep informed of advances in the field.

COMMUNICATION

When other department managers and you meet to discuss new techniques or problems, take a representative from your department with you. Your staff members are frequently more aware of conflicts with their work than you are. Including them also strengthens the team effort concept.

Have formal, documented inservice programs for all changes in techniques, supplies, or work routines. Encourage questions and discussion to prevent misunderstandings. Regular department meetings should be conducted to share any information about the department or things that might affect the department. Encourage employees to share any information, problems, or concerns they might have about the department. In this way you can "iron out" wrinkles and attempt to create a closely knit department.

EMPLOYEE PERFORMANCE AND REVIEW

Develop job descriptions and, when possible, create position levels. The levels may be based on responsibilities, education, kind of work, etc. This provides incentive for employees and supplies management with a basis for recognizing exceptional employee performance.

Keep complete and accurate records of the performance of each employee and discuss all entries with him or her. Performances that meet or exceed expectations should be commended and encouragement given. The reason for a less-than-satisfactory performance should be clarified and help offered to correct the problem. These records should be maintained for the duration of employment and retained for the periods dictated by law. Usually the personnel department will have printed guidelines.

BUDGETING

Budgeting, which is a part of every manager's responsibility, is a way of putting a dollar value on your plans. Anticipated revenues and expenditures are determined by considering the following:

1. Volume of work
2. Hours of work
3. Materials
4. Equipment
5. Historical records
6. Future plans
7. Outside services

The two most common systems of budgeting are "grass-roots budgeting" and "zero base budgeting." The system used is usually dictated by the hospital or clinic. Most books on management discuss budgeting in detail (see Bibliography).

SUMMARY

The preceding discussion pertains to phlebotomy units that are part of a hospital or clinic; the details will vary depending on the size and type of institution. A phlebotomy unit that is not part of a hospital or clinic will require the same basic management, although there will be fewer departments with which to coordinate your work. Usually there will be less variety of specimens collected and fewer STAT requests. It will also be necessary to arrange to have a physician available and to have a plan to care for patients who become ill or have adverse reactions. Otherwise, the rules and requirements remain the same.

REVIEW QUESTIONS

1. True or false: The public's opinion of the clinical laboratory is often based on their treatment by the phlebotomy department. _____

2. How may a computer system be used in phlebotomy units? _____

3. For what type of patient is a soundproof room recommended for phlebotomy? _____

4. To determine the amount of time needed to complete a test or procedure, managers use _____ .

5. Each phlebotomy department should have well-developed _____ and _____ .

Bibliography

Becan-McBride K: Textbook of Clinical Laboratory Supervision. New York, Appleton-Century-Crofts, 1982.

College of American Pathologists: Laboratory Workload Recording Methods. Skokie, IL, College of American Pathologists, 1980.

College of American Pathologists: So You're Going to Collect a Blood Specimen—An Introduction to Phlebotomy. 3rd ed. Danville, IL, College of American Pathologists, 1986.

National Committee for Clinical Laboratory Standards: NCCLS Approved Standard: ASH-3 Standard Procedures for the Collection of Diagnostic Blood Specimens by Venipuncture. Villanova, PA, NCCLS, 1991.

Snyder JR, Senhauser DA: Administration and Supervision in Laboratory Medicine. 2nd ed. Philadelphia, JB Lippincott, 1989.

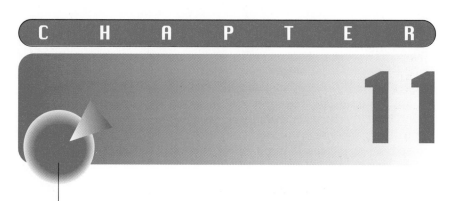

Total Quality in Phlebotomy Service

Mary P. Nix and Maryann D. Harrison

Surviving in today's consumer-oriented market has prompted many organizations to include as part of their mission statement the word "quality": quality products, quality services, quality staff, quality materials. These organizations are committed to quality, as evidenced by the frequently used slogan "customer satisfaction guaranteed." A significant amount of time and resources are spent on ensuring and improving quality, but the benefits—employee satisfaction, improved production, improved teamwork, improved operations, increased market share, increased sales, increased profitability and respect—become vital to an organization's success.

The health care industry, wanting to retain a competitive advantage in business, adopted the practice of ensuring quality. Furthermore, with the changing health care environment and the emergence of managed care and capitation, the health care industry has shifted its focus from mainly quality assurance to continuous quality improvement and outcome measures. Leaders in the health care industry have also included in their mission statements the word "quality." Commitment to, enthusiasm about, and concern for quality patient care—along with market share— equate with success.

The purpose of this chapter is to heighten awareness about quality, to present the principles of quality control, assurance and improvement, and to apply them to phlebotomy.

QUALITY: DEFINITION AND PRINCIPLES

What is quality? To strive for quality, it is important to know what it is. **Quality** is best defined as a degree of excellence. This definition tends to be most applicable not only to businesses, but also to society-wide issues.

The principles of quality in business lie in fact and perception. Doing the right thing, doing it the right way, doing it right the first time, and doing it on time all are aspects of quality. These aspects of quality, when applied to the health care setting, are often driven by outside agencies, both government (e.g., Food and Drug Administration [FDA]) and voluntary accrediting agencies (e.g., Joint Commission on the Accreditation of Healthcare Organizations [JCAHO]).

The perceptions of quality include delivering the right product, satisfying the customer's needs, meeting the customer's expectations, and treating every customer with integrity, courtesy, and respect. Even if the aspects of quality are met, will they alone be enough to attract and retain customers?

Achieving balance between the aspects and perceptions of quality requires constant adjusting. Xerox, Federal Express, and Motorola, Inc.

are examples of quality award-winning companies. These and others serve as role models for many health care-oriented businesses.

QUALITY CONTROL

Clinical laboratory scientists performed quality work and provided quality results long before the term "quality assurance" became popular. How? By performing quality control. **Quality control (QC)** is the process that validates final results and quantifies variations. When a test (e.g., glucose) is performed on a patient specimen, control samples representing high, low, and normal results are also tested. Decisions about the reportability of the patient's results are made based on a comparison with the results of the control testing. Quality control enables laboratory scientists to confidently report accurate and reproducible test results. In phlebotomy, QC relates to ensuring that correct criteria for specimen integrity are met. These include heating or icing specimens, determining that patient preparation is appropriate (e.g., fasting for glucose tolerance test), and accuracy of timed draws.

If clinical laboratory practitioners have a close association with quality already, why the increased attention to ensuring it? In addition to economic survival, the pressures of external forces such as accrediting agencies, government regulations, and the public have increased. Since the mid-to-late 1980s, every health care organization has been striving to provide high-quality, cost-effective patient care. What has changed over the years is the increased emphasis on customer satisfaction.

QUALITY ASSURANCE

Quality Assurance (QA), to the health care practitioner, is the process of making sure that standards of care have been maintained. The use of laboratory tests to diagnose disease and monitor treatments has significantly increased over time, resulting in a proportionate increase in the importance of ensuring overall laboratory quality. QA takes on a broad view, unlike QC, which is specific (e.g., test or product related). Assuring quality in the laboratory means assessing the entire department's operation to identify areas with negative outcomes and those with positive outcomes (e.g., staff, procedures, training, QC, equipment, computers, and materials/supplies). This is accomplished by establishing **indicators** (i.e., specific, measurable variables) and **thresholds** (i.e., points/values prompting study of an aspect of care), collecting and analyzing data, taking **corrective action,** and monitoring the effectiveness of the corrective action, and reporting this information to the appropriate personnel.

QC then becomes a part of a QA program. It is possible to have a QC program without having a QA program; this is how laboratories operated for many years. However, it is not possible to have a QA program without QC.

QUALITY IMPROVEMENT

Quality Improvement (QI) is the constant search for ways to improve product, service, and performance. This can be seen in examples such as the emphasis now on making health care services easier to access, or friendlier, as in "one stop shopping." The transition to safer products like latex-free tourniquets and gloves, and safer medical devices like needles designed to prevent needlestick injury are additional examples of searching for excellence (quality). Consider the use of bar-coded labels in the laboratory to increase efficiency and reliability as another example.

A major component of QI is performance, such as the phlebotomist's responsiveness to patient's concerns, satisfaction, and the quality of care given. There is a continuous effort to heighten phlebotomists' awareness and sensitivity through a variety of mechanisms, e.g., feedback from, patient surveys and continuing education programs.

A well-directed quality program will enable one to see the components of an operation that need to be corrected to meet and adhere to the standards of care. Just as important, a well-directed program enables one to see the components of an operation that are already high in quality, efficient, and cost-effective (i.e., not requiring corrective action). Many times the need to improve an aspect of care for one section of a health care facility requires interdepartmental involvement and teamwork. Anticipated benefits from this type of activity are significant improvement in the quality of care delivered by that facility, and increased satisfaction.

The following quality tools can be found in a facility that has quality care, and improvement, as its focus:

1. Information important to decision making is communicated (usually by memorandum, newsletter, staff meetings, or logbook).

2. Orientation and training are well structured (not too long, not too short, and with checklists pertaining to important aspects of the job).

3. Continuing education is strongly encouraged, and ideally, provided.

4. Respect and caring are promoted.

5. Performance is monitored by supervisory personnel and compared with standards (not with the performance of coworkers), and appraisals conducted.

6. Standard operating procedure (SOP) manuals are up-to-date, written by supervisory personnel citing accrediting and governing agencies' regulations when necessary, reviewed by the director annually, and serve as a reference for all employees.

7. Each employee has a personnel file on record containing items of no surprise to the employee (e.g., job description, performance evaluations, counseling documentation, letters of commendation, etc.).

8. Proficiency/competency tests are distributed to the staff on a rotational basis or given to all staff when sufficient quantity exists to do so.

9. Individual participation in scheduled quality activities are included in the job description.

10. Equipment and instruments are calibrated, maintained, and serviced as scheduled.

11. Computer systems are validated before use and monitored thereafter.

12. The workplace and environment are safe.

13. There are leaders who actively seek suggestions and communicate objectives.

14. Documentation of all of these items is expected (Table 11–1).

TABLE 11-1 • Tools for Assuring Quality

---

1. Active two-way communication
2. Well-structured orientation and training
3. Periodic continuing education
4. Promotion of respect and caring
5. Monitored and appraised performance
6. Standard operating procedure manuals
7. Accurate personnel file
8. Periodic proficiency/competency testing
9. Participation in QC and QA activities
10. Properly functioning and maintained equipment and supplies
11. Validated and monitored computer systems
12. Safe work environment
13. Leaders who seek suggestions
14. Documentation

Additional information about these items can be found in Chapters 9 and 10. As you may be able to see, quality improvement expands on the foundations of quality control and quality assurance, needs to be organization-wide, seems daunting at times, and is inevitably never-ending.

ASPECTS OF QUALITY IN PHLEBOTOMY SERVICE

Performing the right type of phlebotomy (venipuncture vs. skin puncture), doing it the right way (i.e., per procedure), doing it correctly the first time, and doing it on time are the aspects of quality in phlebotomy. Many of these aspects have already been detailed elsewhere in this textbook. Adhering to these procedures is one step toward quality patient care.

The importance of ensuring quality in phlebotomy is best stated this way: "A test result is no better than the quality of the specimen received in the laboratory."[1] Having quality technicians/technologists, quality procedures, and quality instrumentation means little if the specimen received in the laboratory is of poor quality. Specimens of low quality can produce inaccurate and potentially dangerous results. This may have a negative and possibly expensive outcome on patient care: the wrong treatment may be administered, the wrong patient may be treated, the wrong dosage may be given, the wrong blood type may be transfused, and patient death may even occur as a consequence of an improperly collected specimen. Obviously both the patient and the health care facility want to avoid these situations. Phlebotomists directly affect these pre-analytic variables and should strive for quality in their work so that these negative outcomes can be avoided.

Because blood and other body fluids begin to change immediately after collection from the body, the specimen collector should be trained to take steps that will minimize these changes. These steps include the following:

1. Using and referring to clearly written procedures.
2. Ensuring the completeness and accuracy of information on requisition forms.
3. Using the correct collection technique and tube types.
4. Meeting all specimen and labeling requirements.
5. Transporting the specimen to the laboratory according to procedure.

The laboratory that performs the tests is responsible for preparing the procedure manuals and other important information regarding procurement of blood or body fluid specimens. This information should be provided to every health care professional involved in the phlebotomy process. Adherence to these steps ensures that the specimen, and ultimately the test result, will be an accurate reflection of the patient's condition and lead to a positive patient outcome.

THE PROCEDURE MANUAL FOR SPECIMEN COLLECTION

The most important step in ensuring quality phlebotomy is using and referring to the procedures that describe, outline, and detail specimen collection. Table 11–2 summarizes the contents of specimen collection manuals useful in ensuring quality blood specimens.

Professionals are not expected to remember all of the details in the procedure manual. However, they should know its general content, where to readily locate it, and remember that the manual exists for their reference. It contains answers for most specimen-related questions and should be used when the patient's life is not in jeopardy.

It is our experience that most phlebotomy errors occur because standard operating procedures are not followed. After the training period, when a question comes to mind, the specimen collection manual should be consulted for the answer. In the hospital setting, all nursing units should have a specimen collection manual, as nurses, medical students, and physicians sometimes procure specimens. Therefore, the manual should be accessible to them, as well as to the phlebotomist, at all times. The laboratory supervisor should be contacted when the procedure is unclear, thought to be outdated, or difficult to find.

TABLE 11–2 • Specimen Collection Manual: Contents Useful in Assuring Quality Specimens

1. The following should be included for each test:
   a. Test name and alternative name(s)
   b. Patient preparation
   c. Type of specimen
   d. Timing requirements
   e. Type of tube/container
   f. Transportation requirements
   g. Labeling requirements
   h. Test requisition form or code
   i. Name and telephone number of laboratory
2. Criteria for unacceptable specimens
3. Steps for handling inability to collect specimen
4. Requirements for acceptable newborn/pediatric samples

Each test performed in the laboratory is addressed in the specimen collection manual. The test name, including alternative names, notes on how to prepare the patient for the test (e.g., fasting), the type of preferred specimen (e.g., venous), notes on timing requirements (e.g., for glucose tolerance tests), and the type of container in which to collect the specimen (e.g., EDTA Vacutainer tube) should be included. Transportation requirements emphasizing the effects of time, temperature, exposure to light, and excessive vibration or rough handling can be found in this manual. Adherence to these requirements is critical to certain tests (e.g., bilirubin). Adherence to specimen labeling requirements is also critical for some tests, especially those performed by the blood bank; therefore, labeling procedures are included in the manual.[2] Figure 11–1, a sample page from an existing manual, illustrates many of these items.

The appropriate test requisition form and the name of the laboratory performing the test can be found in the manual, along with the laboratory's telephone number. Interestingly, the test requisition form may be another, more practical source of specimen collection information. As shown in Figure 11–2, many of the items found in the collection manual are also found on the test requisition form. In a computerized facility, where computerized labels are used, in lieu of requisitions, this information can be found on the computer label.

Unacceptable Specimens. Some specimen collection manuals also include, for each test, the criteria for an unacceptable specimen. Specimen rejection may occur, for example, when (1) labeling is inadequate or improper; (2) collection is not timely (e.g., within a certain number of hours after treatment); (3) the sample volume is insufficient for the test being ordered, especially when the specimen container includes an additive; (4) the wrong collection tube or container is used; (5) a collection tube is used after its expiration date; (6) the sample is transported incorrectly (e.g., not sent on ice); and (7) the specimen is found to be hemolyzed (which can adversely affect tests such as potassium). When a specimen is deemed to be unacceptable, it usually must be recollected. Unacceptable specimens, recollected specimens, and duplicate specimen collections are central to the phlebotomy quality process.

Unsuccessful Collection Attempts. In addition to unacceptable specimen criteria, the specimen collection manual should include a procedure listing the steps the phlebotomist can take when unable to collect a blood specimen. This procedure should address unsuccessful venipunctures, patient unavailability, and patient refusal to be tested. In each scenario, documentation (see Fig. 11–3) is important for quality review, as the problem must be identified and corrected. Therefore, the number of collection attempts is included as an indicator in the phlebotomy quality program.

TEST	SPECIMEN INSTRUCTIONS	HP*	REFERENCE RANGE	CODE	FEE
BETA-SUBUNIT PREGNANCY TESTS - See HCG listings.					
BETA - 2 MICROGLOBULIN, SERUM	3 mL blood, red top tube.		20-39 yr: 0-2.0 mg/L 40-59 yr: 0-2.6 60-79 yr: 0-3.1	B2M	64.00
BETA -2 MICROGLOBULIN, URINE (Referral Lab)	10 mL urine, random specimen.		5-154 mcg/L	B2UR	32.00
BILIRUBIN, TOTAL AND DIRECT	2 mL blood, red top tube.		Total: 0.2-1.2 mg/dL Direct: 0.0-0.4	BIL	37.00
BILIRUBIN, TOTAL MICRO (NEONATAL BILIRUBIN)	Blood; 1 red or green Microtainer. Protect from light.			MBL	84.00
BIOPSY - See Surgical Pathology.					
BLASTOMYOCOSIS ANTIBODY	5 mL blood, red top tube. Consultation with lab suggested (955-6363). Fill out Microbiology request and case history form.			BLY	134.00
NOTE: Antibody to blastomyces may be significant when interpreted in light of a suggestive clinical picture. CF titers of 1:8 are also suggestive. Higher titers or rising titers are more significant.					
BLASTOMYOCOSIS CULTURE (Referral Lab)	7-10 mL blood, isolator tube.				
BLEEDING TIME (TEMPLATE)	Performed Monday-Friday on day shift. Schedule with lab 1 day in advance (955-7687).		2-8 Minutes	BT	84.00

*HP: Highest lab priority available (S=Stat, A=ASAP)

FIGURE 11-1 • Sample page from a laboratory specimen collection manual. (From Laboratory Information Handbook. Philadelphia, Thomas Jefferson University Hospital Clinical Laboratories, October, 1998, p. 30.)

THOMAS JEFFERSON UNIVERSITY HOSPITAL
CLINICAL LABORATORIES
DIRECTOR: FRED GORSTEIN, M.D.

OUTPATIENT ONLY - *PLEASE PRINT*

PATIENT'S NAME - LAST | FIRST | SEX | DATE OF BIRTH

☐ **EMERGENCY** ☐ PHONE ☐ FAX _____ (SPECIFY WHICH)

STREET ADDRESS

NOTE: STAT SPECIMENS MUST BE BROUGHT DIRECTLY TO LAB (3RD FLOOR, PAVILION)

CITY | STATE | ZIP CODE

SPECIMEN COLLECTED (REQUIRED BY STATE LAW) | DATE | TIME ☐ AM ☐ PM

PHYSICIAN ORDERING TEST - LAST NAME | FIRST

NAME OF COLLECTOR

STREET ADDRESS

MEDICATION
☐ COUMADIN ☐ HEPARIN ☐ ASPIRIN ☐ OTHER _____

CITY | STATE | ZIP CODE

ICD-9 CODE:

SPECIMEN MUST BE LABELED WITH PATIENT'S NAME

USE ADDRESSOPLATE OR PRINT THE ABOVE

(TO SPECIFY COMMON ICD-9 CODES, SEE REVERSE)
ORDER CANNOT BE BE PROCESSED WITHOUT DIAGNOSIS
To the Physician: Clinical consultants from the laboratory are available to help in the selection of appropriate tests.
Call 215 955-6545 or -6381.

SPECIMEN NOTES (SEE REVERSE)

SPECIMEN NOTES (SEE REVERSE) | SPECIMEN NOTES (SEE REVERSE) | SPECIMEN NOTES (SEE REVERSE)

CHEMISTRY TEST GROUPS

BLOOD

☐ SM7 BASIC METABOLIC PANEL(80049) R5
☐ CO2 CARBON DIOXIDE (82374) R2
☐ CL CHLORIDE (82435) R2
☐ CRT CREATININE (82565) R2
☐ GLF GLUCOSE (82947) R2 1
☐ K POTASSIUM (84132) R2
☐ NA SODIUM (84295) R2
☐ BUN UREA-N (84520) R2
☐ MCM COMPREHENSIVE (80054) R5
    METABOLIC PANEL
☐ ALB ALBUMIN (82040) R2
☐ TBIL BILIRUBIN, TOTAL (82250) R2
☐ CA CALCIUM (82310) R2
☐ CL CHLORIDE (82435) R2
☐ CRT CREATININE (82565) R2
☐ GLF GLUCOSE (82947) R2 1
☐ ALP ALKALINE (84075) R2
    PHOSPHATASE
☐ K POTASSIUM (84132) R2
☐ PRO PROTEIN, TOTAL (84155) R2
☐ NA SODIUM (84295) R2
☐ AST AST (SGOT) (84450) R2
☐ BUN UREA-N (84520) R2
☐ ELC ELECTROLYTES (80051) R5
☐ CO2 CARBON DIOXIDE (82374) R2
☐ CL CHLORIDE (82435) R2
☐ K POTASSIUM (84132) R2
☐ NA SODIUM (84295) R2
☐ HPM HEPATIC (80058) R5
    FUNCTION PANEL
☐ ALB ALBUMIN (82040) R2
☐ BIL BILIRUBIN, (82251) R2
    TOTAL AND DIRECT
☐ ALP ALKALINE (84075) R2
    PHOSPHATASE
☐ AST AST (SGOT) (84450) R2
☐ ALT ALT (SGPT) (84460) R2
☐ CRK LIPID PANEL (80061) R5 1,9
☐ COL CHOLESTEROL (82465) R2 1,9
☐ HDL HDL-CHOLESTEROL (83718) R5 1,9
☐ GLC TRIGLYCERIDES (84478) R2 1,9

NON-FDA APPROVED TESTS: Medicare will not provide reimbursement for tests which are not approved by the FDA for patient care. These include, among others: CA 15-9, P24 Antigen, Cyclosporine (Non-Specific), Erythropoietin, etc. In addition, Medicare will not provide reimbursement for tests ordered for screening purposes only.
(1) This test includes interpretation; if interpretation is not required, please circle test name.
(2) If the initial result for this test is positive, the laboratory will automatically perform normal and usual follow-on test(s). If you do not want the Laboratory to perform these test(s), or require that your advance approval be obtained, please circle the test name, and write in your instructions.

☐ ACN ACETONE (82010) R1
☐ ACPR ACID PHOSPHATASE (84060) R3 11
☐ ACT ACTH (82024) L3 11
☐ AP2 AFP+2 (TRIPLE SCREEN) R10
    (82105, 84233, 84702)
☐ MA MICROALBUMIN (82043) UR
☐ ALO ALCOHOL, ETHYL (82055) R5
☐ ATN ALDOSTERONE (82088) R2
☐ APN ALPHA FETOPROTEIN (1) (82105) R5
    MATERNAL SCREENING
☐ APM ALPHA FETOPROTEIN (82105) R5
    TUMOR MARKER
☐ AML AMYLASE (82150) R2
☐ AND ANDROSTENEDIONE (82157) R2
☐ ACE ANGIOTENSIN (82164) R2
    CONVERTING ENZYME
☐ DNA ANTI dsDNA AB (86225) R5
☐ ANA ANTINUCLEAR AB (86038) R5
☐ ATA ANTI-THYROID ABS (86800) R5
☐ CGF HCG, BLOOD (84702) R2
    FULL TITER
☐ MBL BILIRUBIN, NEONATAL (82250) 12
☐ CAO CA 125 (86316) R2
☐ CAI CALCIUM, IONIZED (82330) G5 11
☐ CEA CEA (82378) R2
☐ CPK CK (82550) R2
☐ C34 COMPLEMENT (C3, C4) (86160) R2
☐ CBC CBC WITH PLATELETS (85029) L3 2
    (NO DIFF)
☐ CBA CBC W/DIFF & PLT (85025, 85023) L3
☐ PTR PATHOLOGIST REVIEW 10
    OF BLOOD SMEAR
☐ COR CORTISOL (82533) R2
☐ CLS CYCLOSPORINE (80158) L3 3
☐ DHE DHEA-S (82627) R2
☐ DIG DIGOXIN (80162) R2
☐ DIL DILANTIN (80185) R2
☐ EST ESTRADIOL-17B (82670) R5
☐ FER FERRITIN (82728) R2
☐ FOA FOLATE (82746) R2
☐ FSH FSH (83001) R2
☐ GGT GGT (82977) R2
☐ GLH GLYCOHEMOGLOBIN (83036) L5
☐ HGE HEMOGLOBIN (1) (83020) L2
    ELECTROPHORESIS
☐ HPA HEP A AB PROFILE (1) (86296) R3 4
☐ HBC HEP B CORE AB (1) (86289) R2
☐ HBS HEP B SURF AB (1) (86291) R2
☐ HAA HEP B SURF AG (1) (86287) R2
☐ HPC HEPATITIS C AB (86302) R3
☐ IGE IMMUNOGLOBULIN-E (82785) R2
☐ IME IMMUNOFIXATION (84165, 86320) R4
    ELECTROPHORESIS (1)

☐ IMG IMMUNOGLOBULINS (86329) R2
    QUANTITATIVE
☐ IIB IRON+IRON (83540, 83550) R5
    BINDING
☐ LDH LD (83615) R2
☐ LH LH (83002) R2
☐ LSE LIPASE (83690) R2
☐ LTH LITHIUM (80178) R2
☐ DRVT LUPUS INHIB (85613) B3
☐ LYA LYME ANTIBODY (86618) R5
☐ MG MAGNESIUM (83735) R2
☐ FTA FTA TREPONEMA (86781) R10
☐ MNO MONONUCLEOSIS (86308) R5
    SCREEN
☐ OSM OSMOLALITY (83930) R1
☐ PHE PHENOBARBITAL (80184) R2
☐ PHO PHOS PHATE (84100) R2
☐ PRG PROGESTERONE (84144) R2
☐ PCN PROLACTIN (84146) R2
☐ PSAS PROSTATE SPECIFIC (84153) R3
    ANTIGEN
☐ PRE PROTEIN (1) (84165) R3 5
    ELECTROPHORESIS
☐ PT PROTHROMBIN TIME (85610) B3 6
☐ PTT PTT [PARTIAL, (65730) B3 6
    THROMBOPLASTIN
    TIME (ACTIVITY)]
☐ PTH PTH, INTACT, (83970) R5
    (INCL CALCIUM)
☐ RPR RAPID PLASMA REAGIN (86592) R5
☐ REN RENIN ACTIVITY (84244) L5
☐ RTC RETICULOCYTES (85045) L2
☐ RHF RHEUMATOID FACTOR (86430) R5
☐ RUB RUBELLA SCREEN (86762) R5
☐ SED SED RATE (85651) K5
☐ SIK SICKLE CELL (85660) L2
☐ T3R T3 TOTAL (84481) R2
☐ T3U T3 UPTAKE (84479) R2 7
☐ FT4 FREE T4 (84439) R2
☐ T4R T4 (84436) R2 7
☐ T7 T7 (84479, 84436) R2
☐ TEG TEGRETOL (80156) R2
☐ FTS TESTOSTERONE (84402) R3
    FREE AND TOTAL
☐ TES TESTOSTERONE, TOTAL (84403) R2
☐ THE THEOPHYLLINE (80198) R2
☐ TFR TRANSFERRIN (84466) R1
☐ TSH TSH(THYROID SCREEN) (84443) R2 8
☐ URC URATE (84550) R2
☐ VAL VALPROIC ACID (80184) R2
☐ B12 VITAMIN B12 (82607) R2

URINE

☐ CGI HCG(QUAL) (84703) UR
☐ UCA CALCIUM (82340) UT
☐ UCR CREATININE (82570) UT

☐ UCC CREATININE CLEARANCE(82575) R2 UT
☐ UOS OSMOLALITY (83935) UR
☐ UPR PROTEIN (84155) UT
☐ UEL PROTEIN (1) (84155) UT
    ELECTROPHORESIS
☐ UMAC URINALYSIS (2) (81003) UR
    MACROSCOPE ONLY
☐ UA URINALYSIS, (81001) UR
    INCL MICROSCOPIC
☐ VMA VMA (84585) U24 14

OTHER FLUIDS

☐ SFG GLUCOSE, CSF (82947) C1
☐ SFP PROTEIN, CSF (84155) C1

OTHER TESTS - WRITE IN

_____
_____
_____
_____
_____

URINE TIMES

	MON	DAY	TIME
BEGUN			☐ AM ☐ PM
ENDED			☐ AM ☐ PM

LAB USE ONLY
TOTAL TIME _____ HR
VOLUME _____ ML

BLUE BACKGROUND - AVAILABLE AS STAT PROCEDURE

BILLING INFORMATION - REVERSE P.2

LAB USE ONLY
ACCO. NO. _____

_____
_____
_____

LAB I.D. _____

★★SPECIMEN INFORMATION - SEE REVERSE★★

0466-01 (4/98)

PATIENT MUST READ AND SIGN STATEMENT ON REVERSE OF FORM.

FIGURE 11-2 • Sample test requisition form. (Courtesy of Thomas Jefferson University Hospital Clinical Laboratories, Philadelphia, PA.)

SPECIMEN NOTES

1. Fasting specimen.
2. Consists of WBC, RBC, HGB, HCT MCV, MCH, MCHC, RDW and Platelets (Quant)
3. Submit whole blood only.
4. Profile includes IgG and IgM
5. Includes Protein Electrophoresis and Total Protein.
6. Tube must contain 2.7 mL (in 3 mL Hemogard Blue Top Tube).
7. If T3 Uptake and T4 are both ordered, T7 will be calculated by the lab.

8. TSH is the recommended Thyroid screening test.
9. If all 3 components of the Lipid Panel are ordered, LDL-Cholesterol is calculated.
10. CBA order is required.
11. Collect on ice.
12. Protect from light.
13. Heparinized whole blood; rush to lab on ice.
14. Collect with 4 Boric Acid tablets.

SPECIMEN TYPE AND AMOUNT

A - ARTERIAL
AF - AMNIOTIC FLUID
B - BLUE TOP TUBE (ALWAYS FILL TUBE)
C - CEREBRO SPINAL FLUID
G - GREEN TOP TUBE
K - BLACK TOP TUBE (ALWAYS FILL TUBE)
L - LAVENDER TOP TUBE
M - MICROTAINER

R - RED TOP TUBE
GAST - GASTRIC CONTENT
UR - URINE, RANDOM SAMPLE
UT - URINE, TIMED COLLECTION
U24 - URINE, 24 HOUR COLLECTION

(FOR UT AND U24 - INDICATE "BEGIN" AND "ENDED" TIMES IN "URINE TIMES" BOX ON FRONT OF FORM)

LABORATORY INFORMATION 955-6545
MICROBIOLOGY USE LAB FORM 0473-01
CYTOLOGY USE LAB FORM 0476-00
FLOW CYTOMETRY USE LAB FORM 0489-00
HIV TESTING USE LAB FORM 0473-02

NUMBER FOLLOWING THE SPECIMEN OR TUBE CODE ON THE FRONT OF THIS FORM INDICATES THE MINIMUM AMOUNT OF SPECIMEN TO BE DRAWN, IN ML. FOR EXAMPLE, R5 REPRESENTS 5 ML BLOOD IN A RED TUBE

COMMON ICD9 (DIAGNOSIS) CODES - CHECK ALL THAT APPLY The codes listed are some of the frequently used diagnosis codes and are provided for convenience only. It is the physician's responsibility to assign the most appropriate and specific diagnosis code for the tests ordered, and it may be necessary to consult the current ICD-9-CM manual for additional, more specific, or more appropriate codes.

Code	Description	Code	Description	Code	Description	Code	Description
78900	Abdomen Pain Unspec Site ___	3056	Cocaine abuse ___	075	Infectious mononucleosis ___	29534	Paran Schizo-Othr/Exacerb ___
7890	Abdominal pain ___	30580	Cocaine Abuse Unspec ___	5699	Intestinal disorder NOS ___	29532	Paranoid schizo-chronic ___
64880	Abn Glucose in Preg-Unsp ___	30480	Comb Drug Dep NEC-Unspec ___	129	Intestinal Parasitism Unspec ___	486	Pneumonia, organism NOS ___
7945	ABN Thyroid func. Study ___	2860	Coag Factor VIII Disord ___	984	Lead, Toxic Effect ___	9583	Posttraum Wnd Infec NEC ___
7919	Abn Urine Findings Nec ___	4280	Congestive Heart Failure ___	2729	Lipid metabol. Dis NOS ___	V222	Pregnancy State, Incidental ___
7832	Abnormal loss of weight ___	920	Contusion Face/Scalp/Nck ___	5739	Liver Disorder NOS ___	6029	Prostate Disorder NOS ___
6360	Absence of menstruation ___	7803	Convulsions ___	V427	Liver transplant status ___	2989	Psychosis NOS ___
30300	Ac alcohol intox-unspec ___	4140	Coronary Atherosclerosis ___	1628	Mal Neo Bronch/Lung NEC ___	2720	Pure Hypercholesterolem ___
3030	Ac Alcohol intoxication ___	7862	Cough ___	1729	Malig melanoma skin NOS ___	59080	Pyelonephritis NOS ___
7061	Acne NEC ___	4644	Croup ___	1916	Malig Neo Brain NEC ___	7806	Pyrexia Unknown origin ___
462	Acute Pharyngitis ___	5959	Cystitis NOS ___	1919	Malig Neo Brain NEC ___	5939	Renal and Ureteral Dis NOS ___
4619	Acute Sinusitis, Unspecified ___	2963	Depr Psych, Recur Episod ___	1869	Melig Neo Testis NEC ___	5199	Resp System Disease NOS ___
4659	Acute URI NOS ___	29620	Depress Psychosis-Unspec ___	1748	Malign Neopl Breast NEC ___	78609	Respiratory abnorm NEC ___
30928	ADJ React mixed emotion ___	311	Depressive Disorder NEC ___	185	Malign Neopl Prostate ___	7140	Rheumatoid Arthritis ___
3099	Adjustment reaction NOS ___	2500	Diabetes Mellitus Uncomp. ___	1539	Malignant Neo Colon-NOS ___	V700	Routine Medical Exam ___
30500	Alcohol Abuse- Unspec ___	2469	Disorder of thyroid NOS ___	1538	Malignant Neo Colon NEC ___	29572	Schizoaffective-Chronic ___
2859	Anemia NOS ___	7804	Dizziness and Giddiness ___	1749	Malignant Neopl breast NOS ___	29570	Schizoaffective-Unspec ___
V289	Antenatal Screening NOS ___	30590	Drug Abuse NEC-Unspec ___	1541	Malignant neopl Rectum ___	29590	Schizophrenia NOS-Unspec ___
30000	Anxiety State, NOS ___	3059	Drug Abuse NEC/NOS ___	V703	Med Exam NEC-Admin Purp ___	V789	Scree-Blood Dis NOS ___
71690	Arthropathy NOS- Unspec ___	304.9	Drug dependence, Unspec ___	6268	Menstrual disorder NEC ___	282.6	Sickle Cell Anemia ___
49390	Asthma w/o status asthm ___	2929	Drug mental disorder NOS ___	632	Missed abortion ___	8470	Sprain of neck ___
42731	Atrial fibrillation ___	995.2	Drug Substance, Adverse Effect ___	075	Mononucleosis, Infectious ___	V252	Sterilization ___
040	Bacterial Diseases, other ___	6339	Ectopic Pregnancy NOS ___	340	Multiple sclerosis ___	5369	Stomach function dis NOS ___
4011	Benign Hypertension ___	79093	Elevated PSA (Prostate) ___	3009	Neurotic Disorder NOS ___	0340	Strep sore Throat ___
2967	Bipolar affective NOS ___	2599	Endocrine Disorder NOS ___	25000	NIDDM w/o complication ___	V221	Supervis Oth normal preg ___
2984	Bipolar Affective, Manic ___	34590	Epilep NOS w/o intrac EP ___	768.43	Nocturia ___	7802	Syncope and collapse ___
2899	Blood disease NOS ___	6149	Fem Pelv Inflam Dis NOS ___	5589	Noninf Gastroenterit NEC ___	7100	Syst Lupus Erythematosus ___
30183	Borderline personality ___	V708	General Medical Exam NEC ___	6236	Noninflam dis vagina NEC ___	64003	Threat Abort Antepar COM ___
85400	Brain Injury NEC ___	7809	General symptoms NEC ___	7821	Nonspecif skin erupt NEC ___	24290	Thyrotox NOS No Crisis ___
3090	Brief Depressive React ___	2409	Goiter NOS ___	2410	Nontox Uninodular goiter ___	130	Toxoplasmosis ___
490	Bronchitis NOS ___	V723	Gynecologic examination ___	V22	Normal pregnancy ___	13101	Trichomonal vaginitis ___
2349	CA in Situ NOS ___	7840	Headache ___	278	Obesity ___	59780	Urethritis NOS ___
5920	Calculus of kidney ___	4299	Heart Disease NOS ___	V715	Observ following rape ___	5990	Urine Tract Infection NOS ___
1121	Candidal vulvovaginitis ___	5997	Hematuria ___	V718	Observ-Suspect Cond NEC ___	7589	Urinary Sys Symptom NEC ___
6180	Cervicitis ___	054	Herpes Simplex ___	30401	Opioid dependence-Contin ___	6161	Vaginitis ___
75249	Cervix / Fem Gen Anom NEC ___	042	HIV ___	73300	Osteoporosis NOS ___	61610	Vaginitis NOS ___
78659	Chest pain NEC ___	5733	Hepatitis, unspecified ___	116	Opportunistic Mycoses ___	0999	Venereal Disease NOS ___
78650	Chest pain NOS ___	2724	Hyperlipidemia NEC/NOS ___	65370	Oth Abn Fet Disprop-UNSP ___	0068	Viral enteritis NOS ___
496	Chr Airway Obstruct NEC ___	600	Hyperplasia of prostate ___	V5849	Other Spec Surg Aftercare ___	0796	Viral/Chlamydi Infec NOS ___
585	Chronic Renal Failure ___	4019	Hypertension NOS ___	6202	Ovarian Cyst NEC/NOS ___	070	Viral Hepatitis ___
4739	Chronic sinusitis NOS ___	2449	Hypothyroidism ___	7295	Pain in Limb ___		
2869	Coagul Defect NEC/NOS ___	009	Ill defined intestinal infection ___	7851	Palpitations ___	NEC: Not Elsewhere Classifiable
						NOS: Not otherwise specified	

FIGURE 11-2 • *Continued* Reverse side of form.

UNCOLLECTED SPECIMEN NOTICE THOMAS JEFFERSON UNIVERSITY HOSPITAL CLINICAL LABORATORIES	ROOM No.

PATIENT'S NAME

TEST(S)

Specimens requested were not collected because:

☐ Patient not in room - Call Lab to re-schedule

☐ Patient uncooperative _____

☐ Unable to draw _____

☐ Other: _____

COLLECTOR	TIME ☐a.m. ☐p.m.	DATE

LA-T-1

FIGURE 11-3 • Sample uncollected specimen notice. (From Laboratory Information Handbook. Philadelphia, Thomas Jefferson University Hospital Clinical Laboratories, October, 1998, p. 9.)

Newborn and Pediatric Patients. Finally, the unique handling of newborn and pediatric patients should be covered in the specimen collection procedure manual. Specifically, the minimum amount of blood needed to perform a laboratory test on one of these patients should be highlighted in the manual. An example of pediatric specimen requirements is shown in Figure 11–4. Many premature infants undergo transfusion merely to replace blood removed for laboratory testing (known as iatrogenic blood loss). By collecting the smallest amount of blood required for testing, significant blood loss can be avoided. Because of the small blood volumes in newborns and children, the number of times blood is collected and the amounts removed from these patients should be monitored and included in the phlebotomy quality program.

QUALITY CONTROL OF SUPPLIES AND INSTRUMENTS

The best QA & QI and practices in phlebotomy depend on the phlebotomists who are trained to perform blood collection procedures. Reports from phlebotomists that evacuated tubes are not working properly (e.g., not drawing the appropriate amount) may result in the performance of a blood collection QC procedure. The implementation of a new brand of tube or of a modified evacuated tube may also be reason to perform a QC procedure.

Blood collection QC procedures may or may not be included in a phlebotomy QA program, depending on the particular facility's interests and experiences. If difficulties are encountered by the workers who use

CAPILLARY SPECIMEN REQUIREMENTS

Pediatric specimens are accepted for a number of tests. This section lists all the common ones for which pediatric specimens can be used, and indicates the number of Microtainer blood tubes which are needed. This list is classified by general test type, i.e., chemistry, hematology, and so forth. Most specimens are serum (red top Microtainer), however please note that some require EDTA (lavender top tube).

Specimen amounts indicated apply where the hematocrit of the patient is normal. If the hematocrit is high, it is suggested that the amounts shown be doubled.

	NUMBER of MICROTAINER(S)	COLOR
CHEMISTRY		
Acid Phosphatase	2	Red/Green
Albumin	1/3	Red/Green
Alkaline Phosphatase	2/3	Red/Green
ALT	2/3	Red/Green
Amylase	1/3	Red/Green
AST	2/3	Red/Green
Bilirubin (Fractionated)	1/2	Red/Green
Calcium	1/3	Red/Green
Chem-7 Panel (SMA7)	1	Red/Green
Chloride	1/3	Red/Green
Cholesterol	1/3	Red/Green
CO_2	1/3	Red/Green
Complement C3, C4	1	Red
CK	2/3	Red/Green
CK Isoenzymes	1	Red
Creatinine	1/3	Red/Green
Enzymes	1	Red
GGT	2/3	Red/Green
Glucose	1/3	Red/Green
Health Screen-12 (SMA 12)	1	Red/Green
Hemoglobin, Plasma Free	1	Lavender
Immunoelectrophoresis	1	Red
Immunoglobulins	1	Red
LD	2/3	Red/Green
LD Isoenzymes	1	Red
Lipase	1	Red/Green
Magnesium	1/3	Red/Green
Microbilirubin	1/2	Red/Green
Osmolality	2/3	Red/Green
Phosphate	1/3	Red/Green
Potassium	1/3	Red/Green
Protein Electrophoresis	1	Red
Protein, Total	1/3	Red/Green
Sodium	1/3	Red/Green
Total Protein	1/3	Red/Green

FIGURE 11-4 • Sample pediatric specimen requirements. (From Laboratory Information Handbook. Philadelphia, Thomas Jefferson University Hospital Clinical Laboratories, October, 1998, p. 100.)

TABLE 11-3 • Phlebotomy QC Procedures

1. Evaluation of evacuated test tubes
2. Evaluation of stopper assembly
3. Centrifuge test
4. Additive test

---

the vacuum tubes, or if new technologies are implemented, the supplier or manufacturer may be contacted and asked to assist with corrective action or provide consultation.

Whether performed by the laboratory or by the manufacturer, phlebotomy QC may include one of the four procedures listed in Table 11–3 and discussed in the text that follows.

Evaluating Evacuated Test Tubes. The purpose of evaluating evacuated test tubes is to measure the amount of vacuum draw and compare it with expected results under standard test conditions. A 1-m piece of flexible vinyl or latex tubing is connected to the tip of a 50-ml buret. A 20-gauge blood collection needle is attached to the open end of the tubing. The procedure continues by filling the buret with water, bleeding the air out of the tubing and needle, refilling the buret to bring the meniscus to "0," inserting the needle into the stopper of an evacuated tube, opening the stopcock of the buret, pushing the needle through the stopper, and allowing the tube to draw completely. The tube is then elevated so that its meniscus is at the same height as the buret meniscus (Fig. 11–5). The stopcock is closed, and the volume drawn from the buret is recorded (to 0.1 ml). Each tube for which the tested draw does not fall within ±10% of the labeled draw is defective.

Evaluating the Stopper Assembly. The purpose of evaluating the stopper assembly is to ensure that it will function as expected during collection and sample mixing. Evacuated vacuum tubes are filled with water using a 20-gauge blood collection needle and holder. While the tube is removed slowly from the needle/holder, the stopper is examined to make sure it does not pull out of the tube. After placing the tube in a mechanical mixer and mixing for 20 minutes, the stopper is observed for overall looseness and leakage of water at the puncture point or around the tube's rim. Stoppers that pull out, fall out, have general looseness, or leak during the steps of this test procedure are defective.

Centrifuge Test. In the centrifuge test, the ability of an evacuated tube to withstand the centrifugation needed to separate whole blood into its components is evaluated. After the vacuum tubes are completely filled with water, they are placed in centrifuge carriers, following the centrifuge manufacturer's directions. The tubes are spun for 10 minutes with a 2200 relative centrifugal force. Tube breakage of any degree indicates a defect.

Additive Test. The additive assay determines the quantity and identity of the chemical (e.g., anticoagulant) added to the evacuated tube. Assays follow United States Pharmacopeia (USP) or other appropriate chemical methods.

VACUUM DRAW

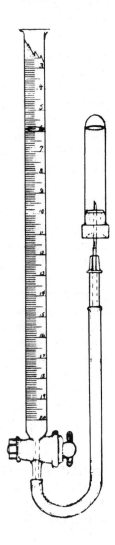

FIGURE 11-5 • Method for evaluating the amount of vacuum draw in evacuated test tubes. (Reproduced with permission from H1-A4, "Evacuated Tubes and Additives for Blood Specimen Collection—Fourth Edition; Approved Standard," NCCLS, 940 West Valley Road, Suite 1400, Wayne, PA 19087, U.S.A., 1996.)

More detailed instructions for any of these QC procedures can be obtained from the National Committee for Clinical Laboratory Standards (NCCLS)[3] (771 East Lancaster Avenue, Villanova, PA 19085; telephone, (610) 525-2435).

PERCEPTIONS OF QUALITY IN PHLEBOTOMY SERVICE

Delivering the right product/service (e.g., collection of blood specimens); satisfying the customer's needs and concerns; meeting the customer's expectations; and treating every customer with integrity, courtesy, respect, and care directly affect the perceptions of quality in phlebotomy. Who are the customers of a phlebotomist? Patients are not the only customers; the patient's family, doctors, nurses, and other departments' employees are also customers.

What are the needs of these customers? Regardless of the customer, the need is assistance in detecting or treating an illness and professional service. All customers expect a relatively painless venipuncture, proper timing, clear instructions, use of proper technique, adherence to standard operating procedure (consistency), efficiency, effective interpersonal communication skills, and teamwork. Customers do not want or expect additional stresses. They want to be treated with integrity, courtesy, and respect. Using the best venipuncture technique means nothing to the customer who has been mistreated (e.g., yelled at, forced or coerced to permit testing, lied to, given false hopes, made the recipient of prejudice, etc.). Professional behavior is a key to quality patient care.

It is important to remember that phlebotomists are usually the only representative of the clinical laboratory who have direct patient contact. Patients, doctors, nurses, and others who have had an unpleasant experience with a phlebotomist are likely to have a negative image of the laboratory and its ability to provide quality services. However, the converse is also true. Positive experiences tend to yield positive patient outcomes. Members of a phlebotomy team can be considered the laboratory's public relations officers. Therefore, a laboratory quality monitoring program might include customer satisfaction surveys and incident report monitoring.

At times, extraneous situations arise that can interfere with quality work. Examples include, but are not limited to, patients who are being resuscitated, patients with traumatic injuries, combative patients, uncooperative family members, belligerent doctors or nurses, and frequent experiences of heavy workload and low staffing. Each of these, or any combination, tend to be stressful for the phlebotomist.

When these extraneous situations occur, effective coping tactics are needed. "All employees need to short-circuit negative emotions, especially anger, and achieve a level of calmness, clarity, and peace that lets them perform at their best."[4] Maintaining focus, adhering to standard operating procedures and referring to the manual when questioned, practicing assertive behaviors (neither aggressive nor passive), being empathetic, and displaying a caring professional image will enable phlebotomists to handle these stressful occasions with pride and a positive outcome.

SUMMARY

A phlebotomy total quality program is designed by combining the technical aspects of blood collection and the customers' perceptions of quality of service with regulatory requirements for monitoring, evaluating, and continuously improving service. Positive patient outcomes are the goal of any health care delivery service. Using and referring to the procedures in the specimen collection manual and reporting problems to supervisory personnel are important to assuring quality. The number and types of specimens rejected, the number of specimens recollected, the number of duplicate draws, the number of collection attempts, the number of specimens drawn from newborn and pediatric patients, incidents of untimeliness, and cases of customer complaints are usually the indicators included in the phlebotomy quality plan. Factors contributing to poor quality services are sought and analyzed; corrective action is taken, when indicated; and the effectiveness of this action is studied. The search for ways to maintain quality standards, keep costs down, retain existing customers, and attract new customers are crucial to survival in today's marketplace.

Each employee's involvement in the entire process is fundamental to successful QC, QA, and QI plans. Monitoring and evaluating quality is a time-consuming process. However, the benefits (positive outcomes, satisfied customers, improved teamwork, improved profitability and market share, etc.) are worth the investment, and are important to an organization's success.

REVIEW QUESTIONS

1. The document with which every phlebotomist must be familiar is the _____ .
2. Evaluating vacuum tubes is a form of phlebotomy _____ .

3. Customer _____ surveys are part of monitoring programs.

4. Quality _____ is the focus of health care organizations.
5. The process of monitoring, evaluating, and correcting patient care problems is called quality _____ .

References

1. Hunt VD: Quality in America: How to Implement a Competitive Quality Program. Homewood, IL, Business One Irwin, 1992.
2. Stewart CE, Koepke JA: Basic Quality Assurance Practices for Clinical Laboratories. Philadelphia, JB Lippincott, 1987, p 17.
3. National Committee for Clinical Laboratory Standards: Evacuated Tubes for Blood Specimen Collection. 3rd ed. Document H1-A3. Villanova, PA, NCCLS, 1991.
4. McCutchen G: Total quality people. *Clin Lab Sci,* 5:94–95, 1992.

Bibliography

American Association of Blood Banks: Accreditation Requirement Manual. Bethesda, MD, American Association of Blood Banks, 1996.
College of American Pathologists, Commission on Laboratory Accreditation: General Laboratory Inspection Checklist. Northfield, IL, CAP, 1996.
Joint Commission on Accreditation of Healthcare Organizations: 1996 Comprehensive Accreditation Manual for Pathology and Clinical Laboratory Services. Oakbrook Terrace, IL, JCAHO, 1996.

Medical-Legal Issues and Health Law Procedures

Shirley E. Greening

213

The term medical–legal describes the interrelationship of the professions of law and medicine. The medical–legal field is sometimes called "medical law" or "legal medicine." Early medical law most often concentrated on forensic medicine, or the presentation of medical data or evidence in courts of law. Medical law has now expanded to encompass such fields as pathology, psychiatry, toxicology, public health regulation, health care legislation, court rulings, and administrative regulation of medical professional practice and medical service programs. Health law is a specialty area of law that relates to practitioners in medicine, dentistry, nursing, hospital administration, environmental health and safety, and allied health. The allied health professions include those individuals who work in laboratories located in hospitals, public health facilities, private or commercial enterprises, and research settings.[1]

Phlebotomists, as members of the laboratory health care team, are in a unique position in relation to most other laboratory personnel. In many health care settings phlebotomists may be the only laboratorians who come into face-to-face contact with patients or blood donors; they are the only laboratorians who perform specimen collection procedures on patients or donors, and the only laboratorians who deal with the very real issues of fear of infection, illness, and death and dying from the patient's perspective. Phlebotomists must have a strong educational background and good training; be technically proficient; follow laboratory procedures; be in compliance with government rules and regulations; and at the same time be good listeners, good communicators, and good public relations representatives. If phlebotomists become inattentive to, careless about, or unaware of their professional roles and duties, they may increase the risk of errors in the practice of their profession and thus increase the risk of being held legally liable for those errors. Examples of the most common errors are injury to a blood donor, misidentification of a patient, a mistake in interpreting a physician's orders, and transmission of disease.

Phlebotomists practice their profession at a time when patients and clients have high expectations for the success of their health care. Patients and clients are increasingly likely to question the quality of care or to object to treatments or procedures that they have perceived as harmful, injurious, or damaging to them. One result of this questioning may be that the patient or client takes legal action by filing a malpractice **claim** against the health care institution, the laboratory, and any individuals involved in their care, including phlebotomists.[2,3]

Another result may be that government regulatory agencies or laboratory accreditation organizations may call into question the way that a laboratory supervises its personnel or the ways in which a laboratory ensures that it is providing quality services and care to patients and clients.

Phlebotomists should be familiar with the various legal principles and the regulatory framework that affect their activities as members of the health care team. Phlebotomists should not conduct their professional activities in constant fear of legal liability (what some have termed "defensive medicine"). Rather, an understanding of why and how medical–legal issues arise in the day-to-day performance of phlebotomists' duties is part of phlebotomy education and practice.

SOURCES OF LAWS

Common law consists of those principles and rules of action that derive their authority solely from usages and customs that have evolved from ancient, unwritten laws of England. The common law is all the statutory and case law background of England and the American colonies before the American Revolution and is distinguished from statutory or legislative law, which developed after the American Revolution. Many common law principles have been incorporated into more formalized bodies of law governing cities, states, and nations.

Statutory law (also called "legislative law") is the body of law that is developed and promulgated by the United States Congress or by a state legislature as an outcome of the political process or societal influences.

Legislatively enacted laws are called "statutes." A municipality may also enact laws, which are usually called "codes" or "ordinances."

Administrative law (also called "regulatory law") is not technically a set of laws, but instead consists of the rules and regulations that are written by government agencies to implement statutes or public laws. The United States Congress delegates authority to a variety of government agencies that then write the specific provisions of the statutes in a process know as **rulemaking.** Most agencies also have the power to monitor compliance with these rules and enforce penalties for noncompliance. In contrast to courts or legislatures, government agencies employ and consult with experts having special knowledge about the areas covered by statutes. Agencies also have much greater flexibility than courts or legislatures to revise regulations in response to social and economic changes or new scientific information. Courts or legislatures may defer to a government agency for an interpretation of a court rule or legislative statute.[4]

Decisional law (also called "case law") develops as a result of federal, state, or local courts deciding cases brought by two or more individual parties. Cases are decided based on precedents (a decision in a previous case), which can then be narrowed, expanded, distinguished, or overruled. Case law that is decided "once and for all" is termed *stare decisis;* if an issue had been litigated before by the same parties and cannot be litigated again, it is termed *res judicata.*[5] Case law can become statutory law where local, state, or federal government legislatures vote to incorporate a judicial line of decisions into the form of a statute. By passing legislation, governments recognize that decisions in individual cases have importance and application to all citizens.

Each source of law or method of law-making (statutory, case, and administrative) may deal with civil laws, criminal laws, or laws of equity. *Civil laws* are those that relate to private rights and remedies sought by citizens through proceedings termed civil actions. Civil actions are brought to enforce, redress, or protect an individual's private rights. *Criminal laws* (also termed "penal laws") refer to those state and federal statutes that define criminal offenses and specify corresponding penalties, fines, and punishments for offenses against the safety and welfare of the public or wrongs committed against the federal government or a state government. Criminal laws generally apply to misconduct that is willful, intentional, wanton, or reckless. The doctrine of *equity* was developed to administer justice on principles of fairness, especially when a court or an administrative agency does not have the power or the legal precedents to make, carry out, or enforce a decision.

Standards of proof in cases brought before regulatory, civil, or criminal forums are variable and can overlap depending on the severity and extent of a violation. For example, most questions regarding regulatory law are decided based on whether there was substantial compliance with an agency's rule or regulation. In a civil action, a plaintiff must show that it was more probable than not that a defendant caused an injury or other type of harm. Most criminal cases require that evidence of guilt be beyond a reasonable doubt.

AREAS OF LAW APPLICABLE TO PHLEBOTOMY PRACTICE

The phlebotomist's interactions with patients, clients, and other health care professionals can be viewed from different legal perspectives. Health care workers (most commonly physicians) and patients could be viewed as having an implied contractual relationship. A contract is formed when the physician offers or makes available health services, and the patient agrees to the medical care. The contract is formalized when the physician is paid. There is no requirement for an express written agreement between these two parties to the contract—the actions undertaken by the physician and patient essentially imply that a contract has been made. However, the physician–patient relationship thus formed is more than a mere business deal; it is a voluntary arrangement most aptly seen as creating a status or relationship rather than a contract. The physician-patient relationship gives rise to certain professional duties and **fiduciary** obligations even when there is no payment for services.[6]

A physician or a patient could be in breach of contract if either does not meet his or her part of the agreement. However, it is rare indeed for a physician to take legal action against a patient for not following medical instructions. In health law, it is overwhelmingly the patient who sues a physician, hospital, or health care worker. Why do patients sue? Because they believe the health professional has failed to do something that he or she should have done. This failure to meet a **standard of care,** when the health professional has a duty of due care to a patient, most commonly falls under the area of law known as torts. For a variety of reasons, claims against health care personnel are usually framed in terms of tortious conduct rather than breach of contract. Patients do not claim that a physician or other health care worker violated a contract; they claim that he or she committed a tort.[7]

A tort (from the Latin word *torquere,* meaning twisted) is a civil wrong or injury, other than breach of contract, that may be remedied by a court in the form of an action for damages. All torts involve a violation of some duty that is owed by one individual to another individual. When phlebotomists, a phlebotomy service, or a laboratory employing phlebotomists is held liable for an injury or other damage to a patient or client, each may be blamed for intentionally or unintentionally acting, or failing to act, in a manner that caused an injury. The patient or client who claims to be injured is called the **plaintiff.** The person being blamed is the **defendant.**

INTENTIONAL TORTS

In the context of health care, claims falling under the category of intentional torts usually arise in conjunction with questions about whether a patient gave permission for or consented to a medical procedure, a treatment, or a diagnostic test. When these circumstances occur, they are generally framed as a charge of *assault* or *battery*. In most jurisdictions, assault and battery are criminal offenses.

Assault is any active, willful attempt or threat to inflict injury on another person that is coupled with an apparent ability to inflict such harm. Assault can be committed without actually touching or striking; it is the plaintiff's sense of awareness and apprehension of imminent harm that determines whether there is an assault. Assault is often defined as an unlawful attempt to commit a battery.

Battery can be viewed as an active intent to cause harm or injury to a person without that person's consent that actually does harm the person. The offer or threat to use harm is an assault; the use of it is battery. Because battery always includes an assault, the two are commonly combined in the phrase "assault and battery." The term "technical battery" is sometimes used to describe those situations in which a physician or other health care worker, in the course of treatment, exceeds the consent given by the patient even though no harmful purpose was intended.

When a patient enters a hospital or a client comes into a blood-drawing center, the presumption is that he or she has consented to be treated or has consented to be a donor. However, few individuals would give blanket consent to any and all possible medical procedures without being given more information with which to make an informed choice. (See "Consent and Informed Consent.") If a phlebotomist proceeds to collect blood after a patient has refused to have blood drawn, the patient could claim that the act of the phlebotomist approaching him or her with a needle was an assault. If the act of drawing blood was perceived by the patient as painful or injurious, he or she could claim that a battery was committed.

It is not uncommon for patients to feel stress when confronted with medical decisions and procedures. However, occasionally the behavior of health care personnel can intentionally or unintentionally produce severe emotional reactions in patients. Intentional behavior (conduct or words) that is particularly outrageous and extreme can lead to a charge of intentional infliction of emotional distress. Even if conduct is not intended to threaten, if the patient perceives a threat, he or she may claim negligent infliction of emotional distress. Obviously, the phlebotomist must avoid threatening language ("if you don't let me draw blood, you're going to die") or gestures (acting out a painful procedure) that could create such distress.

UNINTENTIONAL TORTS

When a health care worker violates a duty owed to a patient or client, it is called "malpractice." Malpractice can be defined as professional misconduct, an unreasonable lack of skill in or faithfulness to professional duties, illegal or immoral conduct, ignorance, or neglectful or careless mistreatment that leads to injury, unnecessary suffering, or death of a patient or client. Most legal actions involving malpractice by health care personnel are grounded in the theory of **negligence,** the failure of a "duty of due care."

Negligence: What Must Be Proved?

In every legal action for negligence, the plaintiff must go through a four-step process to prove that a health care worker is at fault for failing to perform some legal duty. These four steps, called "elements," are duty, breach of duty, causation, and damages.

Plaintiffs have the burden of proving each of these four elements. In most malpractice cases, if even one element cannot be proved, then the defendant is not held liable for malpractice. However, in some instances an average reasonable person who has no special professional knowledge could conclude that an injury would not have occurred in the absence of a negligent act. When a breach of duty is obvious to a layperson, the doctrine of *res ipsa loquitur* ("the thing speaks for itself") can be applied. This has the effect of shifting the **burden of proof** to the defendant, who must then prove that he or she was *not* negligent.

Duty. As a citizen, every individual has a duty to behave as a reasonably careful person would, given the same or similar circumstances. This standard of behavior means that individuals must act or refrain from acting so as not to injure or damage another person or that person's property. The duty to meet a standard of behavior or care can arise from a state statute or city ordinance (e.g., "Do not cross the street when the light is red"). In health care, duty is usually established by standards of care or practice that exist by custom or by professional rules and guidelines. The legal standard of care is " . . . that degree of skill, proficiency, knowledge and care ordinarily possessed and employed by members in the profession . . . " The standard has to be shown to exist, and the phlebotomist must be performing in the capacity applicable to that standard.

Those persons engaged in professions that require special knowledge and skills are judged according to a standard of care upheld by similar professionals. For the phlebotomist, the test to determine what he or she did or should have done would be, "What would a reasonable, prudent phlebotomist have done under the same or similar circumstances?" In the past, physicians and other health professionals were held to standards that existed in their own communities (the so-called locality rule). Because health professionals now have access to information outside of their own communities, this standard has been expanded to include what would be expected in similar communities. When national standards exist, such as national certification examinations or national accreditation standards for schools, a national standard of care can be imposed. This is true for the profession of phlebotomy—for example, a phlebotomist in California would be held to the same standard of care used for a phlebotomist in New York.

Breach of Duty. Conduct that exposes others to an unreasonable risk of harm is a breach of duty. The plaintiff must be able to show what actually happened and that the defendant acted unreasonably. Either **direct** or **circumstantial evidence** can demonstrate what happened. If the defendant knew or should have known that there was a reasonable probability that his or her conduct would cause harm, then the defendant will be found to have breached the duty of due care.

Causation. The cause of harm or injury is both a factual and a legal question. To show *cause-in-fact* (or actual cause), the plaintiff must demonstrate that he or she would not have been injured but for the conduct of the defendant. There must be a direct line from the conduct to the injury, with no intervening circumstances and no other factors or events that contributed to the injury. "Proximate cause" is the term used to distinguish legal causation from factual causation. Legal (proximate) cause is a policy choice that essentially determines who should bear the costs of harm. If an injury was reasonably foreseeable by the defendant, then the defendant will be held legally liable for the injury.

Damages. Once negligence and causation are established, plaintiffs must be able to show that they were actually damaged by the negligent act. The harm to a plaintiff may be physical, emotional, or financial. In these circumstances, courts attempt to place a monetary value on the injury. Compensatory damages attempt to reimburse the plaintiff to the position the plaintiff was in before he or she was injured. Special damages allow recovery of economic losses during the time of injury, which may be for medical bills or lost wages, but can also be for future losses. Future losses might include the costs of continuing medical treatment or loss of future wages if the person is unable to return to work. General damages are those costs related to the injury itself. Punitive damages, those assessed to punish a defendant, are usually not awarded in negligence cases, unless the defendant's conduct was reckless or willful.

Liability of Employers for Phlebotomy Personnel

Most phlebotomists are employed by hospitals, independent laboratories, or other health care organizations, and when a phlebotomist is found to be negligent, his or her employer can also be found negligent. The employer, employee's supervisor, or a laboratory director may be vicariously liable when the employee's negligent conduct falls within the scope of the employment, regardless of whether the employer was actually present or had the ability to control the employee's conduct. *Respondeat superior* ("let the master answer") is the legal doctrine that places an employer in a position of responsibility for the acts of its employees. An employer has an affirmative duty to control the conduct of employees.

In corporate negligence theory, a hospital, its board of directors, administrators, and reviewing committees, and any other persons who act as agents for the corporation owe a duty of due care to patients. The principles of corporate negligence are similar to those of vicarious liability, but in corporate negligence, liability is imposed on the corporate entity and on nonmedical agents of the corporation, rather than on negligent physicians or allied health personnel. Examples of corporate negligence include a hospital's hiring an unqualified laboratorian, or a hospital's maintaining an unsafe environment for patient treatment.

The types of duties owed by a hospital directly to a patient include a duty to use reasonable care in maintaining safe and adequate equipment and facilities, a duty to oversee all who practice medicine within the hospital walls, a duty to select and retain competent physician and nonphysician personnel, and a duty to establish and enforce policies and rules that ensure quality care for patients.[8] Under corporate liability, a hospital cannot avoid liability by delegating these duties to physicians or other individuals who work in the hospital.

HOW IS THE PHLEBOTOMY STANDARD OF CARE DETERMINED?

Courts and plaintiffs rely on a variety of sources to show that standards of care and practice exist for a particular profession. All states have statutes called "Medical Practice Acts" (MPAs) that define the qualifications and experience necessary to legally practice medicine. MPAs usually delineate which medical procedures or tests can be delegated to other health personnel under a physician's supervision, and they prohibit anyone who is not licensed as a physician or other health professional (such as a nurse or physical therapist) from practicing healing or diagnostic medicine. State licensing boards generally review cases in which a person is engaged in the unauthorized practice of medicine. MPAs are enforced through disciplinary actions imposed by licensing boards and, in extreme cases, by criminal sanctions.[9]

Many states also *license* allied health personnel. Because most state licensing boards require some proof of qualification for licensure, lack of a license may be used to demonstrate a failure to meet a standard of care. Situations may arise in which a person has the appropriate education, training, or experience to practice in an allied health profession but does not have a license to practice. When an individual is not licensed and malpractice is shown, that individual's conduct may be declared to be **negligence per se,** in which practicing without a license is a violation of a statute.[5]

Hospital and laboratory *certification or accreditation standards and guidelines* can be used to demonstrate quality control and quality assurance procedures in phlebotomy practice. Even when standards are voluntary, compliance with or awareness of standards and guidelines can be used to show that a phlebotomy service or a phlebotomist knew or should have known what procedures and conduct were appropriate under the circumstances. Certification and accreditation guidelines are especially effective as **evidence** of practice standards when they are applicable nation-wide and followed by a wide variety and number of phlebotomy services and phlebotomy practitioners. Examples of organizations that accredit or certify phlebotomy services include the Joint Commission on Accreditation of Healthcare Organizations (JCAHO), the College of American Pathologists (CAP), and the American Association of Blood Banks (AABB).

Mandatory standards in the form of federal, state, and local laws and regulations are commonly used to establish a statutory standard of practice for phlebotomy services. Regulations usually outline minimum standards of performance. Mere compliance with a statutory requirement does not necessarily protect phlebotomy services and personnel from negligence actions, especially if it can be shown that personnel knew or should have known that more comprehensive actions were required, either in general or as related to the specific circumstances surrounding the plaintiff. Examples of federal statutory standards are those contained in the Clinical Laboratory Improvement Amendments of 1988 (CLIA '88)[10] and the Occupational Safety and Health Administration's (OSHA's) Rules on Occupational Exposure to Bloodborne Pathogens.[11] States may have health and safety statutes that are similar to or more stringent than federal standards. Cities usually have health and safety codes or ordinances that govern areas such as storage of chemicals and disposal of waste materials. When both federal and state laws or regulations apply to laboratory practice, the laboratories are usually required to abide by whichever of the laws is more stringent.

Statements of competencies, such as those contained in the National Accreditation Agency for Clinical Laboratory Sciences' (NAACLS) Phlebotomy Programs Approval Guide,[12] or designated responsibilities such as those listed in the National Phlebotomy Association (NPA) Guidelines[13] describe tasks and skills required of phlebotomy practitioners. These can be used to show how an individual failed to meet a particular level of performance. For example, if there is a question whether a phlebotomist performed a capillary collection correctly and the competency expects an entry-level phlebotomist to be able to perform the correct procedure for capillary collection, the statement of competency can be used to establish the appropriate standard of care.

Professional practice guidelines, which appear in brochures or bulletins written or endorsed by professional organizations, can be used to show a recommended practice that is viewed by the profession as clinically effective or technically superior. Guidelines may relate to timing of blood collections, collection of patient data, preservation and handling procedures, or follow-up and documentation protocols.

Technical guidelines and standards that describe how to perform a certain test or procedure can be used to show how a phlebotomist was negligent in the collection, handling, or transportation of blood specimens.[14]

Scientific journal and textbooks *(learned treatises)* can be used to demonstrate that knowledge was available to a practitioner at the time of the negligent act, thereby showing what the practitioner should have known or done.

The **testimony** of expert witnesses is commonly used to establish the standard of practice in a health profession. In a case involving a phlebotomist, an experienced phlebotomist, a physician, or a phlebotomy supervisor can be asked to state an opinion on what constitutes acceptable quality control or assurance practices.

OTHER LEGAL DOCTRINES AND AREAS OF LAW APPLICABLE TO PHLEBOTOMY PRACTICE

INTERPLAY AMONG THE RIGHTS OF PRIVACY, CONFIDENTIALITY, AND INFORMED CONSENT

Legal disputes involving intentional and unintentional injury to patients and clients by health care workers have their roots in guaranteed individual rights. These rights have their basis in the United States Constitution and Bill of Rights, regardless of whether they are specifically enumerated in the Constitution. For example, the U.S. Constitution does not mention a right of privacy; however, the United States Supreme Court has recognized that a right of privacy exists and that certain areas of privacy are guaranteed under the Constitution.[7] The right of privacy includes the right to confidentiality, and if this right is waived, consent to the waiver must be informed.

Right of Privacy. An individual's right "to be let alone," recognized in all United States jurisdictions, includes the right to be free of "intrusion upon physical and mental solitude or seclusion" and the right to be free of "public disclosure of private facts."[7] Every health care institution and health care worker has a duty to respect a patient's or client's right of privacy, which includes the privacy and confidentiality of information obtained from the patient/client for purposes of diagnosis, medical records, and public health reporting requirements. If a health care worker conducts tests on or publishes information about a patient/client without that person's consent, the health care worker could be sued for wrongful invasion of privacy, **defamation,** or a variety of other actionable torts.

Confidentiality. Health care workers must be vigilant in keeping information about patients and clients confidential. This is especially true in blood banks, transfusion services, and phlebotomy services, where phlebotomists may have access to information about patients who are human immunodeficiency virus (HIV)–positive, have acquired immunodeficiency syndrome (AIDS) or other sexually transmitted diseases, or who may have medical histories that, if disclosed, might cause undue embarrassment to or prejudice or discrimination against that patient. Phlebotomists and their supervisors should understand that they have a legal duty to keep records, documentation, and laboratory test results confidential. This duty may be waived only if a patient has given express permission for the information to be released, if the patient has sued the institution or its health care personnel, or if the health care worker is specifically obligated to release patient information (e.g., to the Centers for Disease Control and Prevention or other authorized public health department). Even in the last situation, care must be taken to ensure that the confidentiality of patient records and reports cannot be breached while they are being communicated or are in transit.[9]

Consent and Informed Consent. Physicians and other health care workers are required to obtain a patient's consent before performing any invasive or diagnostic procedure. Consent can take a variety of forms (e.g., written agreements, spoken words, implicit actions, or making an appointment for a test). In a nineteenth century case, for example, a plaintiffs failure to object to a vaccine that the defendant was preparing to give to the plaintiff conveyed apparent consent to the injection.[15]

However, to agree to a medical procedure, a patient must first know what he or she is agreeing to. Thus, the doctrine of consent has expanded to include *informed consent,* which emphasizes that health care workers must fully disclose any risks, alternatives, and benefits of a procedure or test so that the patient/client can make an informed decision about whether he or she wants to be treated or tested.[16] "[T]he doctrine of informed consent imposes on a physician, before he subjects his patient to medical treatment, the duty to explain the procedure to the patient and to warn him of any material risks or dangers inherent in or collateral to the therapy, so as to enable the patient to make an intelligent and informed choice about whether or not to undergo such treatment."[17]

The correlate to informed consent is *informed refusal.* Patients may refuse treatment for religious, social, financial, or other reasons, but even in these cases a health care worker may be found negligent for the lack of information given to the patient, if the patient didn't have enough information available to make a reasonable decision to forego treatment.[16]

In general, it is the physician who has the duty to disclose adequate information to a patient. Phlebotomists should be wary of volunteering information to a patient in situations where they do not have the legal or professional authority to do so. These situations may be difficult "judgment calls" for the phlebotomist, as patients often ask phlebotomists questions about their treatment or why they are drawing blood. The phlebotomist should politely refer the patient to his or her physician or charge nurse for these explanations.

PATIENT'S BILL OF RIGHTS

In the early 1970s, the American Hospital Association developed a policy statement for health care institutions and their patients that incorporated and reflected the individual rights guaranteed under the legal doctrines of privacy, informed consent, and confidentiality. Since that time, many hospitals have adopted the *Patient's Bill of Rights* into their policy manuals, and some state legislatures have passed Patient's Bill of Rights statutes.[18]

The *Patient's Bill of Rights* is intended to "promote the interests and well-being of the patients and residents of health care facilities."[1] As such, it enumerates the patient's right to respectful care, to adequate information with which to make an informed decision (or refusal) about his or her care, and to confidentiality in treatment and communication of records about his or her medical care program. In addition, the document affirms a patient's right to information about medical bills and charges, possible involvement in medical research and experimentation, and hospital rules and regulations (see Table 9–2).

MEDICAL DEVICES AND EQUIPMENT FAILURES

Phlebotomists use many pieces of equipment or reagents that are manufactured by medical equipment or pharmaceutical companies and then purchased by the hospital or laboratory from manufacturers, distributors, or retailers. These supplies—whether they be needles, syringes, protective equipment or clothing, chemicals, or blood—may, in unusual situations, be defective or unsafe because of the way they were designed, assembled, or screened, or they may be inherently dangerous even when used under normal conditions. When a patient suffers a needle break during blood drawing, has a violent reaction to a drug, or contracts an infectious disease after use of a product, he or she may sue the manufacturer of that product under various legal theories, including negligence, strict liability in tort, and breach of *implied warranty of merchantability.*

Under negligence theory, plaintiffs must prove that defendants have a duty to conform to certain standards of care in the manufacture of their products and to guard against unreasonable risks. *Strict liability in tort* is imposed when manufacturers are held liable for injuries caused by an unreasonably dangerous or defective product, even if there is no finding of fault. Breach of an implied warranty of merchantability may be found, on the basis that manufacturers or sellers of goods should be obligated to provide consumers with products that are fit for the purpose for which they are being sold.

These legal actions fall under the law of *products liability.* Products liability focuses on the liability of suppliers for defective products that cause physical harm. The defect in question may not be the actual product itself; defects may arise because of inadequate packaging, instructions, or warning labels.[19]

The term "product" implies goods that are sold predominantly in commercial settings. Manufacturer liability for defective health care products has received much professional and legal attention, because health care treatment and diagnostic testing has traditionally been viewed as a service rather than as a product. Especially in the areas of blood transfusions (which may result in HIV transmission) and genetically engineered pharmaceuticals (such as coagulation components), the distinction between products and services has been challenged by plaintiffs who sue blood banks or pharmaceutical companies to recover damages resulting from transmission of infectious diseases.

Because the availability of blood and blood products is of great importance to public health, many states have passed blood shield statutes that exempt blood transfers, blood derivatives, or blood products from the threat of products liability lawsuits and specifically mandate that blood components are to be considered medical services, not goods or products. **Immunity** from legal action thus guarantees an adequate blood supply for use in medical emergencies and treatment of chronic blood-related disorders.

CASE LAW

As the range of health care services has expanded and health care personnel have become more specialized, the reach of malpractice **litigation** is no longer confined to the physician-patient relationship and may include nonmedical personnel as part of the health care team. Although most of the following cases did not specifically involve phlebotomists, the situations can be compared to laboratory and phlebotomy practice. These cases demonstrate how non-physician health care personnel can become involved in lawsuits, and remind phlebotomists of the consequences of poor practice standards and procedures.

Belmon v St. Frances Cabrini Hospital, 427 So2d 541, 544 (LaApp, 1983) [Negligent blood sample collection by a medical technician caused hemorrhage.]

Butler v Louisiana State Board of Education, 331 So2d 192, 196 (LaApp, 1976) [A donor fainted and sustained injuries, and a biology professor was held negligent for not giving students previous instructions on blood drawing and donor care.]

St. Paul Fire and Marine Insurance Co v Prothro, 590 SW2d 35 (Ark App 1979) [Negligent physical therapy procedures caused a patient to develop a *Staphylococcus* infection.]

Simpson v Sisters of Charity of Providence, 588 P2d 4 (Or 1978) [Radiology technician performed a poor-quality radiograph that failed to demonstrate a fracture that subsequently caused paralysis.]

Southeastern Kentucky Baptist Hospital, Inc v Bruce, 539 SW2d 286 (Ky 1976) [Misidentification of a patient led to a surgical procedure on the wrong patient.]

Wood v Miller, 76 P2d 963 (Or 1983) [Negligent use of diathermy equipment burned a patient.]

Favalora v Aetna Casualty and Surety Co, 144 So2d 544 (La App 1962) [A patient fainted and fell, causing injuries; a radiology technician and supervising physician were found negligent for not being alert to and prepared for the patient's condition.]

McCormick v Auret (Ga 1980) [Failure to use sterile equipment during venipuncture led to nerve damage secondary to infection.]

Alessio v Crook, 633 SW2d 770 (Tenn App 1982) [Failure to include an x-ray report in the patient's medical record before patient discharge resulted in more extensive surgery than would have been required had the physician seen the report.]

Variety Children's Hospital v Osle, 292 So2d 382 (Fl App D3 1974) [A surgeon failed to label and separate specimens sent to a pathology laboratory. Because the pathologist was unable to determine which of the two specimens was malignant, removal of both of the patient's breasts was necessary.]

Jeanes v Milner, 428 F2d 598 (Ark 1970) [A 1-month delay in mailing specimens to a laboratory resulted in delayed diagnosis of cancer; if it had been detected promptly and treated, the pain and suffering of the patient could have been lessened.]

Ray v Wagner, 176 NW2d 101 (Minn 1970) [A patient claimed a physician was negligent for failing to timely notify her of her malignancy; the patient was found contributorily negligent for giving the physician incomplete and misleading information about how she could be reached.]

Thor v Boska, 113 Cal Rptr 296 (1974) [A physician's inability to produce medical records after he had been sued for malpractice created an inference of guilt.]

Lauro v Travelers Insurance Company, 262 So2d 787 (La App 1972) [A hospital was not negligent for not using the latest laboratory equipment available, where current standards of care demonstrated that the equipment used was acceptable.]

DEFENSES TO LEGAL CLAIMS

If faced with a lawsuit brought by a patient, the laboratory and the phlebotomist may resort to several defenses to avoid a finding of liability.

STATUTES OF LIMITATION

All states have statutes of limitation that restrict or limit the length of time in which a claimant can file a cause of action after an injury. The purpose of statutes of limitation is twofold; first, they are intended to compel legal actions within a reasonable time so that potential litigants have a fair opportunity to defend themselves while evidence and witnesses are still available.[7] Second, they allow presumably innocent parties to continue their lives and livelihoods without the constant and continuing threat of liability.

In malpractice cases, statutes of limitation can start at several points: at the time of the negligent act, at the time when the injury was discovered; or when the physician-patient relationship ends.

The length of time these statutes run varies from state to state and can be as little as a few months to many years, depending on the cause of action and nature of the injury. Statutes of limitation may also be *tolled* (suspended or stopped temporarily) if, for example, the plaintiff is a child, the defendant is absent from the jurisdiction, or the injury in question has been fraudulently concealed.

CONTRIBUTORY NEGLIGENCE

In rare malpractice situations, a patient's own actions may fall below the standard to which a reasonably prudent patient might be expected to conform. For example, if a patient, during the course of a routine blood collection procedure, unreasonably manipulates or otherwise interferes with the venipuncture to the extent that he or she is injured, and then sues the phlebotomist for the injury, the phlebotomist may raise the affirmative defense of contributory negligence.[20]

In some states, contributory negligence completely bars recovery against the defendant, even if the defendant is found negligent. In other states, a finding of contributory negligence has the effect of reducing the amount of monetary damages against a negligent defendant.

ADEQUATE AND ACCURATE RECORDS AS THE BEST DEFENSE

The importance of detailed, legible, comprehensive record keeping and documentation for laboratory procedures and patient identification cannot be overemphasized. Documentation relating to the laboratory not only is required by federal regulations and accreditation organizations, it is also essential in the legal arena. Legal action against a laboratory rarely takes place at the moment malpractice occurs; claims may be filed years later; and even after a claim is filed, it may be several more years before all evidence is collected in the **discovery** process, and the claim is litigated in court. During this waiting period, memories fade, contemporaneous records may be misfiled or lost, and laboratory personnel change.

Laboratory notations and records should never be altered or changed without documentation of the reasons for the change. Indeed, poorly maintained, sloppy, or altered records may prejudice a jury against a laboratory or health care professional, no matter how well intentioned the change might have been.

A laboratory's or phlebotomist's best defense is the ability to produce witnesses and records that substantiate adherence to acceptable professional standards of practice for documenting identifiable specimen collection, test procedures, test reporting, records storage and archiving procedures, quality control and quality assurance methods, and remedial or corrective actions when laboratory errors occur.[7]

CHAIN OF CUSTODY IN THE CLINICAL LABORATORY

Chain of custody is a rule of legal evidence that requires an authorized person (e.g., police officer, attorney, clinical or forensic testing laboratory, or medical examiner) to account for the location, control, and integrity of a specimen, result, or report at all times. Any break in this chain of custody, from specimen collection to the presentation of test results in a court of law, may suggest that the specimen was tampered with or otherwise altered. If continuous and uninterrupted custody cannot be established, the laboratory specimen may not be admissible as evidence in a legal case.[21]

It is not uncommon for phlebotomists to be called on to collect urine or blood specimens from individuals for the purpose of screening for narcotics, alcohol, or infectious agents. Phlebotomists may also be required to transport specimens that may become evidence in a criminal investigation. To establish each link in the chain of custody, each component step of the specimen testing process (including requisition and report forms) must be documented. Most often this is accomplished by a chain-of-custody form that accompanies the specimen. All individuals who receive, release, or otherwise come into contact with the specimen are required to sign, date, and time-stamp the form to show that the specimen was not tampered with. Phlebotomists or other laboratory workers may be asked to testify about their role in maintaining the chain of custody.

Although the primary purpose of establishing a chain of custody is to ensure that evidence is admissible, the documentation required is not unlike the quality and accuracy-based patient test management provisions of CLIA '88 (see later). In legal cases alleging patient misidentification, lost specimens, or missing reports, laboratories may be required to show not only an unbroken chain of custody, but also that they have complied with the provisions of CLIA '88.

LEGAL AND PROFESSIONAL PROTECTIONS FOR THE PHLEBOTOMIST

The legal doctrines and statutory provisions covered in this chapter focus on the rights and protections available to patients, clients, and donors when faced with substandard or negligent laboratory and phlebotomy practices. Phlebotomists, too, may be concerned about their own exposure to hazardous or infectious agents or about unsafe working conditions. Phlebotomists do have recourse to address these concerns, in addition to bringing unsafe conditions to the attention of their immediate supervisors.

When phlebotomy services are understaffed, phlebotomists are sometimes called on to perform additional tasks that are either beyond the scope of their expertise or increase workloads to the point at which patient care is compromised. Especially in the area of nursing, *Protest of Assignment Forms* are sometimes used as a means to alert supervisors to potentially dangerous practice situations. These forms usually become part of the employee's file and therefore should not be used casually or merely to complain about a short-term situation. They should be used by the phlebotomist only when an extra work assignment is protracted, excessive, clearly unreasonable, and imminently dangerous to the phlebotomist or to his or her patients.

The regulations of the Occupational Safety and Health Administration, and analogous state agencies, are specifically designed to protect the health and safety of employees in the workplace. Phlebotomists should report any hazardous or unsafe materials, conditions, or practices to their supervisor and should be active participants in the formulation of workplace policies to avoid or protect against these situations.

It is generally not necessary for phlebotomists to purchase individual professional liability (malpractice insurance) policies, as most health care employers and institutions cover employees under blanket policies. Phlebotomists should check to see whether they are specifically included in or excluded from the employer's insurance policy and whether their employer's policy is an "occurrence" or "claims-made" policy. Occurrence policies protect employees even at a future date, provided that the policy was in effect at the time when the malpractice incident occurred. A claims-made policy is one that must be continually in force at both the time of the incident and the time the claim is made.

Phlebotomists who are self-employed, either as temporary workers placed in positions through an employment agency, or as independent contractors, may purchase professional liability insurance through several companies that provide individual or group coverage to allied health practitioners. Liability policies usually cover monetary damages for personal injuries up to preset limits and usually include coverage for attorney fees and court costs. Many companies provide legal counsel as part of the coverage.

REGULATION OF LABORATORIES AND LABORATORY PRACTITIONERS

In the past few years, laboratories, laboratory practitioners, and other health care workers have been subject to heightened scrutiny and over sight by state and federal government agencies, both for the protection of the health and welfare of the public and for their own protection. Although state laboratory regulation is quite diverse, federal regulation is intended to apply to virtually all laboratory and health care settings.

CLINICAL LABORATORY IMPROVEMENT AMENDMENTS OF 1988

In October 1988, the U.S. Congress passed Public Law 100-578, CLIA '88, amid a flurry of television and newspaper coverage about some poorly run laboratories that were misdiagnosing or mishandling laboratory tests, and reports of questionable business and payment practices. Congress delegated authority to administer this public law to the Health Care Financing Administration (HCFA). The HCFA, within the U.S. Department of Health and Human Services (DHHS), is the agency that administers the federal government's medical reimbursement and health care payment programs, Medicare and Medicaid.

The federal regulations implementing CLIA '88 went into effect on September 1, 1992. They are intended to ensure the quality and accuracy of laboratory testing by creating a uniform set of provisions governing all laboratories that examine human specimens for the diagnosis, prevention, or treatment of any disease or impairment of, or the assessment of the health of, human beings.[10] Virtually every clinical testing laboratory in the United States, whether in a hospital, a physician office laboratory, or an independent facility, must be certified by the federal government. Facilities that only collect or prepare specimens (or both) or only serve as a mailing service and do not perform testing are not considered laboratories.

Laboratories are subject to inspections by federal and state agencies. Government inspectors or their agents can periodically review laboratory operations to ensure compliance with CLIA '88.

Under CLIA '88, the level of regulatory oversight and performance expectations is dependent on the complexity of a given test procedure, rather than on the location or type of laboratory. All laboratory tests (called "analytes") are categorized as waived, moderately complex, or highly complex, with highly complex testing subject to the most stringent regulations. The level of test complexity is determined by assessing the relative simplicity or difficulty of conducting the test and the relative risk of harm to the patient if the test is performed incorrectly.

The CLIA '88 regulations include provisions for preanalytical, analytical, and postanalytical steps in the testing process. Regulations mandate proficiency testing of laboratories based on the types of test they perform. In addition, laboratories are required to demonstrate and document their quality control and quality assurance procedures, to ensure that patient tests and records are managed appropriately, and to demonstrate that testing personnel have adequate education, training, and experience to perform tests. The focus of the CLIA '88 regulations is on *outcome measures*—laboratories must show that the methods used to test specimens lead to accurate, reliable, quality test results.

Laboratories not meeting the conditions required by the CLIA '88 provisions can be subject to various sanctions and penalties. These range from directed plans of correction to withholding of payment from the Medicare and Medicaid programs for laboratory tests. Laboratories that remain out of compliance with the regulations may be shut down or have substantial monetary fines imposed.

Phlebotomists are responsible for performing many of the pre- and postanalytical steps in the blood testing process. The laboratory's overall performance and its ability to maintain consistent and reproducible quality tests rely in large part on the quality and preservation of specimens collected by the phlebotomist. Therefore, knowledge of and compliance with these provisions can not only contribute to quality patient care, but also provide the phlebotomist and the laboratory with some measure of protection against regulatory sanctions and civil lawsuits.

The following selected provisions of CLIA '88 have special significance to phlebotomists and phlebotomy practice.

Subpart J: Patient Test Management

§493.1101 Condition. Each laboratory performing moderate or high complexity testing, or both, must employ and maintain a system that provides for proper patient preparation; proper specimen collection, identification, preservation, transportation, and processing; and accurate result reporting. This system must ensure optimum patient specimen integrity and positive identification throughout the preanalytic (pre-testing), analytic (testing), and postanalytic (post-testing) processes and must meet the standards of this subpart as they apply to the testing performed.

§493.1103 Standard; Procedures for Specimen Submission and Handling.

(a) The laboratory must have available and follow written policies and procedures for each of the following, if applicable: methods used for preparation of patients; specimen collection; specimen labeling; specimen preservation; conditions for specimen transportation; and specimen processing. Such policies and procedures must ensure positive identification and optimum integrity of patient specimens from the time the specimens are collected until testing has been completed and the results reported.

(c) Oral explanation of instructions to patients for specimen collection, including patient preparation, may be used as a supplement to written instructions where applicable.

§493.1105 Standard; Test Requisition.

The laboratory must perform tests only at the written or electronic request of an authorized person. . . . The laboratory must ensure that the requisition or test authorization includes

(a) The patient's name or other unique identifier;

(b) The name and address or other suitable identifiers of the authorized person requesting the test and, if appropriate, the individual responsible for using the test results or the name and address of the laboratory submitting the specimen, including [the name of] a contact person;

(c) The test(s) to be performed;

(d) The date of specimen collection; . . . and

(f) Any additional information relevant and necessary to a specific test to ensure accurate and timely testing and reporting of results.

§403.1107 Standard; Test Records.

The laboratory must maintain a record system to ensure reliable identification of patient specimens as they are processed and tested to assure that accurate test results are reported. These records must identify the personnel performing the testing procedure. . . . The record system must provide documentation of information, including

(a) The patient's identification number, accession number, or other unique identification of the specimen;

(b) The date and time of specimen receipt into the laboratory;

(c) The condition and disposition of specimens that do not meet the laboratory's criteria for specimen acceptability.

§493.1109 Standard; Test Report.

. . . (a) The laboratory must have adequate systems in place to report results in a timely, accurate, reliable, and confidential manner and to ensure patient confidentiality throughout those parts of the total testing process that are under the laboratory's control. . . .

(e) The results or transcripts of laboratory tests or examinations must be released only to authorized persons or the individual responsible for using the test results.

Subpart K: Quality Control

§493.1201 General Quality Control . . . (b). The laboratory must establish and follow written quality control procedures for monitoring and evaluating the quality of the analytical testing process of each method to ensure the accuracy and reliability of patient test results and reports.

§493.1204 Standard; Facilities. The laboratory must provide the space and environmental conditions necessary for conducting the services offered [including space, ventilation, utilities, and safety precautions for protection against physical hazards and biohazardous materials].

§493.1205 Standard; Test Methods. The laboratory must utilize test methods, equipment, instrumentation, reagents, materials, and supplies that provide accurate and reliable test results and test reports.

§493.1211 Standard; Procedure Manual. (a) A written procedure manual for the performance of all analytical methods used by the laboratory must be readily available and followed by all laboratory personnel.

§493.1215 Standard; Equipment Maintenance and Function Checks. The laboratory must perform equipment maintenance and function checks that include electronic, mechanical, and operational checks necessary for the proper test performance and test result reporting of equipment, instruments, and systems. . . .

§493.1221 Standard; Quality Control Records. The laboratory must document and maintain records of all quality control activities . . . for at least two years. . . . In addition, quality control records for blood and blood products must be maintained for a period not less than five years after processing records have been completed or six months after the latest expiration date, whichever is the later date. . . .

Subpart M: Personnel

§493.1423 Standard; Testing Personnel Qualifications. Each

individual performing moderate complexity testing must

(a) Possess a current license issued by the State in which the laboratory is located, if such licensing is required; . . . and

(4) (i) Have earned a high school diploma or equivalent; and

(ii) [Have documentation of training that ensures the individual has the skills required for proper specimen collection, including patient preparation, if applicable, labeling, handling, preservation or fixation, and processing or preparation; for performing preventive maintenance and troubleshooting . . . ; a working knowledge of reagent stability and storage; and an awareness of factors that influence test results.]

Phlebotomists should note that although their specific duties and functions within their work setting may place them outside the scope of personnel standards for the purposes of federal CLIA '88 regulations, the laws of the state in which their workplace is located may have more specific phlebotomy requirements. Therefore, the personnel standards listed above are intended only to provide a general outline.

Subpart P: Quality Assurance

§493.1701. Each laboratory . . . must establish and follow written poli-

cies and procedures for a comprehensive quality assurance program that is designed to monitor and evaluate the ongoing and overall quality of the total testing process. . . . The laboratory's quality assurance program must evaluate the effectiveness of its policies and procedures; identify and correct problems; assure the accurate, reliable, and prompt reporting of test results; and assure the adequacy and competency of the staff. As necessary, the laboratory must revise policies and procedures based on the results of those evaluations. . . . All quality assurance activities must be documented.[10]

OTHER REGULATORY AGENCIES GOVERNING LABORATORIES AND PHLEBOTOMISTS

Many state and federal laws and agencies govern laboratory practice in some way. Employment practices, wages and salaries, business practices, facilities construction, intra- and interstate transportation of specimens, licensing of personnel, and testing methodology are but a sampling of laboratory-related government oversight activities that affect the clinical laboratory. Although a complete listing of these agencies is beyond the scope of this chapter, listed below are the federal agencies, apart from the Health Care Financing Administration, that have substantial influence on laboratories in the United States.[22,23]

The Occupational Safety and Health Act of 1970 established the *Occupational Safety and Health Administration* (OSHA) within the U.S. Department of Labor. The OSHA is the federal agency that sets rules and regulations covering all aspects of employer and employee safety and health. This agency sets workplace standards and regulates such areas as ventilation; noise; fire and electrical safety; labeling and appropriate precautions for flammables; biologic chemical, and radiation hazards; and safe exposure levels.

The *Food and Drug Administration* (FDA) is responsible for the approval of virtually all medical and diagnostic equipment, devices, pharmaceuticals, reagents, and diagnostic tests before they can be marketed for sale and used in health care settings. The FDA, through its process of premarket approval and its content-labeling requirements, has evaluated the safety, clinical efficacy, and medical need of almost all the testing equipment, reagents, and supplies used by the phlebotomist.

The *Centers for Disease Control and Prevention* (CDC), through its various offices and divisions, serves as a federal resource for developing technical and scientific standards and conducting epidemiologic, health and safety, quality assurance, and health evaluation and proficiency studies and programs.

The *Environmental Protection Agency* (EPA) monitors and enforces regulations for the safe disposal of chemical and other hazardous wastes, including biologic hazards.

The *U.S. Postal Service* has developed regulations covering the safe packaging and transport of human biologic specimens through the mails and requires appropriate warning labels to protect postal workers from potentially hazardous or infectious agents.

Importantly, almost all of these agencies or departments (i.e., OSHA, FDA, CDC, HHS) have some level of oversight over transfusion services and blood banks, in addition to general laboratory oversight.

SUMMARY

The ability to demonstrate sound laboratory management principles and compliance with regulatory provisions, professional accreditation guidelines, and practice standards can provide substantial protection against the threat of litigation. No laboratory or health care worker can be completely protected from lawsuits, but potential liability can be minimized by conscientious and continuous attention to good laboratory practice.

REVIEW QUESTIONS

1. The federal agency responsible for approving and regulating medical devices, pharmaceuticals, and diagnostic test kits is the _FDA_ .

2. The legal responsibility of an employer for the negligent acts of employees is called _Vicarious Liability_ .

3. The legal doctrine of _Informed consent_ requires that a patient must be able to make an intelligent and reasoned decision about whether or not he agrees to a medical procedure or diagnostic test.

4. Imposition of liability on manufacturers for defective blood and blood products falls under the law of _Products liability_ .

5. When a patient who has filed a lawsuit has disregarded a physician's orders or acts unreasonably, thus causing all or part of the injuries sustained, the defendant may use the defense of _Contributory negligence_ .

References

1. Curran WJ, Hall MA, Kaye DH: Health Care Law, Forensic Science, and Public Policy. 4th ed. Boston, Little, Brown, 1990.
2. Peterson RG: Malpractice liability of allied health professionals: Developments in an area of critical concern. *J Allied Health,* 14:363–372, 1985.
3. Oliver R: Legal liability of students and residents in the health care setting. *J Med Educ,* 61:560–561, 1986.
4. Gelhorn E, Boyer BB: Administrative Law and Process: In a Nutshell. 2nd ed. St. Paul, MN, West Publishing, 1981.
5. Black MA: Black's Law Dictionary. 5th ed. (abridged). St. Paul, MN, West Publishing, 1983.

6. Havighurst CC: Health Care Law and Policy: Readings, Notes, and Questions. Westbury, NY, The Foundation Press, 1988.
7. Wadlington W, Waltz JR, Dworkin RB: Law and Medicine: Cases and Materials. Mineola, NY, The Foundation Press, 1980.
8. *Thompson v Nason Hospital*, 591 A2d 703 (Pa 1991).
9. Furrow BR, Johnson SH, Jost TS, Schwartz RL: Health Law: Cases, Materials and Problems. 2nd ed. St. Paul, MN, West Publishing, 1991.
10. Department of Health and Human Services, Health Care Financing Administration, Public Health Service: 42 CFR 405 *et seq,* 57 FR 7002-7186, February 28, 1992.
11. Department of Labor, Occupational Safety and Health Administration: Occupational exposure to bloodborne pathogens. 29 CFR 1910.1030; 56 *FR* 64004-64182, December 6, 1991.
12. National Accrediting Agency for Clinical Laboratory Sciences: Phlebotomy Programs Approval Guide. Chicago, NAACLS 1986.
13. National Phlebotomy Association: Guidelines. Washington, NPA, 1980.
14. National Committee for Clinical Laboratory Standards: Procedures for the Collection of Diagnostic Blood Specimens by Skin Puncture. 2nd ed. Code H4-A2, Villanova, NCCLS, 1986; Collection, Transport, and Preparation of Blood Specimens for Coagulation Testing and Performance of Coagulation Assays. NCCLS Document H21-A. Villanova, NCCLS, 1986; Procedures for the Domestic Handling and Transport of Diagnostic Specimens and Etiologic Agents. 2nd ed. Code H5-A2. Villanova, NCCLS, 1985.
15. *O'Brien v Cunard,* 28 NE 266 (Mass. 1891).
16. Swartz M: The patient who refuses medical treatment: A dilemma for hospitals and physicians. *Am J Law Med,* 11:147–194, 1985. See also *Truman v Thomas,* 611 P2d 902 (Ca 1980).
17. *Sard v Hardy,* 879 A2d 1014 (Md 1977).
18. American Hospital Association: Patient's Bill of Rights. Chicago, AHA, 1973.
19. Shapo MS: Products Liability: Cases and Materials. Mineola, NY, The Foundation Press, 1980.
20. *Smith v McClung,* 161 SE 91 (S. Ct. NC 1931).
21. Chamberlain RT: Chain of custody: Its importance and requirements for clinical laboratory specimens. *Lab Med,* 20:477–480, 1989.
22. Wilcox KR, Baynes TE, Crable JV, et al: Laboratory Management. In Inhorn SL, ed: Quality Assurance Practices for Health Laboratories. Boston, American Public Health Association, 1978.
23. Rose SL: Clinical Laboratory Safety. Philadelphia, JB Lippincott, 1984.

GLOSSARY

Activated Partial Thromboplastin Time / A coagulation test to monitor the factors XII, XI, IX, VIII, X, V, II, and I, often referred to as the intrinsic coagulation system.

Adenosine triphosphate (ATP) / Provides energy for cells and physiological reactions such as muscle contraction.

Adrenals / A pair of ductless endocrine glands located above the kidneys.

Aerobic / Condition requiring the presence of oxygen.

Alveoli / Plural of alveolus; small air sacks in the lung where oxygen and waste products are exchanged with the blood.

Ambulatory / Able to walk; not bedridden.

Anaerobic / Conditions without the presence of oxygen.

Analyte / Substance to be assayed.

Androgen / A hormone stimulating the development of male characteristics.

Antibodies / Glycoproteins produced in response to an antigenic stimulus. Also referred to as immunoglobulins.

Anticoagulants / Substances that prevent coagulation.

Antigens / Substances capable of stimulating immune responses. They combine with antibodies to form complexes. Also referred to as immunogens.

Arrhythmia / Abnormal heart beat.

Artherosclerosis / Condition causing plaque buildup which narrows the vessels that supply the heart with blood.

Attenuated / Made weak; or make less able to cause disease.

Axillary / Pertaining to the armpit.

Basal State / A reference point to which test results are compared.

Blood Gases / Oxygen (O_2) and carbon dioxide (CO_2), monitored if patient has a heart and/or lung disorder.

Burden of Proof / The obligation to affirmatively prove the facts of a disputed issue by the evidence presented.

Bacteremia / The presence of microorganisms in the blood.

Barrier Precautions / Protective clothing and other measures taken to prevent or reduce the chance of exposure to a disease-producing agent.

Capital Equipment / Refers to equipment to be maintained indefinitely. Most institutions will set a minimum price for equipment that

241

anything over that amount will be considered capital equipment and require special permission to purchase.

Carbon Dioxide / A waste product of metabolism consisting of one carbon atom and two oxygen atoms (CO_2), excreted primarily through the lungs.

Cardiac Muscle / The muscle of the heart.

Cartilage / A flexible type of connective tissue that is white or yellow in color.

CBC / Anagram for complete blood count which includes red cell count, white cell count, hemoglobin, hematocrit, mean corpuscular volume (MCV), mean cellular hemoglobin (MCH), mean cellular hemoglobin concentration, and platelet count.

Claim / Demand for money or property, or a demand to assert one's own rights. In malpractice claims, an individual files a cause of action (which states the facts that the person believes give rise to a right to judicial relief) and claims an amount of money (damages) he or she believes will compensate him or her for injury.

Coagulation Factors / A series of proteins that, when activated, will result in clot formation.

Conjunctivitis / Inflammation of the mucous membrane that lines the eyelids.

Convulsions / Involuntary muscular contractions and relaxations; can be caused by stress, hysteria, medication, neural defect, etc.

Coronary Heart Disease / Disease of the heart muscle and/or corresponding circulatory components. See Artherosclerosis.

Corrective Action / An activity geared toward problem resolution.

CPR / Cardiopulmonary resuscitation; combination of artificial respiration and circulation.

Defamation / Holding a person up to ridicule, scorn, contempt, or disrespect, and which tends to injure that person's reputation. Defamation includes libel and slander.

Defendant / The person against whom recovery is sought in a lawsuit. In malpractice, the defendant can be a physician, hospital, allied health practitioner, or other health care provider.

Diabetes Mellitus / Disorder of carbohydrate metabolism due to the lack of insulin, characterized by high blood sugar levels.

Diastole, Diastolic / Part of the heart beat cycle when the heart is in relaxation; normal diastolic range is approximately 60 to 80 mm mercury in healthy young adults.

Differential / A breakdown of the various types of WBCs present in peripheral blood.

Discovery / The methods used to obtain facts and information about a case in order to assist in preparation for trial. In health law, discovery can include oral and written questions, asking for laboratory tests and results, requiring physical examination of patients, collecting medical records and documents, or interviewing witnesses.

Edema / The presence of excessive amount of tissue fluid; may be localized or general.

EDTA / Anagram for the anticoagulant *e*thylene*d*iamino*t*etraacetic *a*cid.

Electrocardiography (EKG or ECG) / Graphic recording of the heart's electrical activity.

Electrolytes / Sodium, Na^+, potassium K^+, CL^- and bicarbonate HCO_3-, monitored in patients with renal and/or respiratory diseases.

Epidemiologic / Factors that determine the frequency of disease and its distribution.

Etiologic / The cause of disease.

Evidence / The facts and information about a case that are known, available, or are collected through the discovery process, and which are used to persuade or convince a judge or jury.

    Direct e. / Evidence in the form of testimony of a witness who actually saw, heard, or touched the subject under question.

    Circumstantial e. / Evidence not based on actual personal knowledge, which show indirectly the facts to be proved.

Expired / As used in the text, synonymous with deceased.

Femoral Vein / The major vein that runs on the upper, inner thigh of mammals.

Fiduciary / A person having a duty to act for another's benefit, and in whose actions is placed another's trust, confidence, and faith.

Forensic Medicine / The application of every area of health care knowledge to the purposes and limits of the law.

Gonads / The sex organs; testes and ovaries.

Hemoglobin / The substance contained in red blood cells that transports oxygen from the lungs to the tissues.

Hematoma / A swelling or collection of blood due to a break in a vessel wall.

Hemolysis / The destruction of red blood cells.

Hemorrhage / Abnormal discharge of blood.

Hemostasis / Balance between the stoppage of blood and the circulation of blood within the blood vessels. This process involves platelets, coagulation factors and other substances such as collagen and epinephrine.

Homeostasis / Arrest of bleeding, thereby maintaining the integrity of the blood vessels and the blood flow.

Hormone / A substance secreted by a gland or organ that acts upon another gland or organ. Examples are estrogen, progesterone, adrenalin, and testosterone.

Hypertension / High blood pressure.

Hypoglycemia / Decreased blood sugar level.

Hypotension / Low blood pressure.

Hypothalamus / Portion of the brain that regulates endocrine function and integrates sympathetic and parasympathetic activities.

Hypovolemia / Decreased volume.

Immunity (legal) / Exemption from duties imposed by a law or from liabilities arising from a law.

Indicators / Specific, measurable variables of important aspects of care.

Infectious / Pertaining to a disease caused by a microorganism that may be transmitted to another person.

Inventory / A list of supplies that is updated as supplies are used.

Jargon / As it is used in a laboratory, terms or expressions that may not be understood by individuals not familiar with a clinical laboratory.

Jugular Vein / Major vein that runs on either side of the trachea. The major venipuncture site in animals.

Lactic Acid / A waste product generated from the breakdown of glycogen during muscle activity.

Larynx / A muscular and cartilaginous structure that houses the vocal cords and provides a passageway for air between the pharynx and trachea.

Litigation / A lawsuit, including all the proceedings occurring before, during, and after a trial.

Lipemia / The presence of an abnormally large amount of lipids (fat) in the circulating blood.

Lymph / Generally a clear, colorless fluid that contains protein, water, and lymphocytes.

Maculopapular / A skin eruption consisting of discolored spots or patches on the skin that are not raised nor depressed, combined with solid, red, raised eruptions that resemble pimples.

Mandible / The bone of the lower jaw.

Mastectomy / Removal of the breast.

Medial Saphenous Vein / A major vein that runs on the inner lower leg of mammals.

Metabolism / Physical and chemical changes of substances within the body.

Multiskilling / Proficient at more than one job or task.

Myasthenia Gravis / Disease characterized by great muscular weakness and progressive fatigability.

Negligence / Failure to do something that a reasonable person would ordinarily have done, or which a reasonable person would not have done. Negligence *per se*—the unexcused violation of a statute.

Neoplasms / Abnormal formation of tissue, producing tumors or growths that are harmful to the host.

Nosocomial / Infections acquired by patients while in the hospital.

Opportunistic Infections / Diseases caused by certain microorganisms that would otherwise be nonpathogenic but, due to an altered physiologic state of the host, are given the opportunity to cause infection.

Osteomyelitis / Inflammation of bone usually caused by a pathogenic organism.

Oxygen / An element that is essential to most forms of plant and animal life.

Palpate / Able to feel or touch.

Pathogen / Microorganism or substance able to produce disease.

Percutaneous / Through the skin.

Permucosal / Through the mucous membranes.

Phagocytosis / The engulfment and destruction of solid materials by a cell.

Phenylalanine / An essential amino acid.

Phlebotomy / The surgical opening of a vein to collect blood.

Pituitary / Endocrine gland located near the base of the brain that secretes several hormones.

Plaintiff / The person who brings a legal action or lawsuit (also called a complainant).

Plasma / The clear fluid that collects at the upper half of a tube of centrifuged blood, consisting of serum and protein substances in solution.

Point-of-Care-Testing / Laboratory tests done at the site of the patient.

Polycthemia Vera / Disease characterized by an increasing number of red blood cells and an increase in total blood volume.

Prophylaxis / Measures taken to prevent disease.

Prothrombin Time (PT) / A coagulation test to monitor the factors VII, X, V, II, and I, often referred to as the extrinsic coagulation system.

Quality / A degree of excellence.

Quality Assurance / The process of making sure standards of care have been maintained by detecting, monitoring, evaluating, and correcting problems affecting patient care.

Quality Control / A process that (1) validates actual results by comparing with expected results and (2) quantifies variations between the two.

Recurrent Tarsal Vein / The vein that runs on the inner surface of the guinea pig lower leg.

Respiration / Act of breathing.

Retrorbital Vein / The vein complex behind the inner portion of the eye.

Rulemaking / The process by which governmental agencies conduct research, consult experts, and draft regulations to implement laws passed by Congress or State legislatures.

Sebaceous Gland / A cutaneous gland that produces oil to lubricate skin or hair.

Septicemia / An infection of the blood; the presence of pathogenic organisms in the blood.

Serum / The clear liquid portion of the blood without its fibrin and corpuscles.

Skeletal Muscle / Also known as voluntary or striated muscle; mainly comprises the muscle we can control.

Smooth Muscle / Also known as involuntary muscle; found primarily in the visceral organs.

Sphygmomanometer / An instrument to measure blood pressure.

Standard of Care / That degree of care, competence, or skill that a reasonably prudent person should exercise in the same or similar circumstance.

Standard Precautions / Safety guidelines that replace universal precautions and used for all patients. Applies to blood, all body fluids, nonintact skin, and mucous membranes.

Stereotype / A fixed image or characterization of one group held by another group.

Subordinate / A person whom you are supervisor over.

Syncope / Fainting.

Systole, Systolic / Part of the heart beat cycle when the heart is in contraction; normal systolic range is approximately 100 to 140 mm mercury in healthy young adults.

Tapped / Entered, penetrated (jargon).

Testimony / Evidence given by a witness under oath.

Threshold / Points/values that prompt the study of an aspect of care.

Thyroid / Endocrine gland that regulates the rates of metabolism and body growth.

Vascular Implant / A metal or plastic device surgically placed from which blood can be removed for sampling.

Waived Test / A low complexity clinical test; does not require special training.

WBC / White blood cell(s).

Animal Phlebotomy

Beth V. Dronson

The purpose of this chapter is to acquaint laboratory personnel and students with basic knowledge of animal venipuncture, blood handling techniques, and common tests performed on animals. Often the most difficult part of animal venipuncture is patient cooperation, so the first section explains animal restraint and various venipuncture sites. The major laboratory species of dog, cat, rabbit, rat, mouse, and guinea pig are included in the discussion. The second section explores proper blood handling techniques, including the effects produced by hemolysis and **lipemia.** Tables at the end of the chapter cover common tests run on laboratory animals as well as the types of tube used and the sample size needed.

247

TECHNIQUES FOR OBTAINING BLOOD SAMPLES FROM ANIMALS

The major laboratory species (dog, cat, rabbit, rat, mouse, and guinea pig) each require different venipuncture techniques. In each species there are multiple sites available for venipuncture depending on the amount of blood needed and the type of testing to be done. Each site requires a different restraint technique, often involving an assistant. However, certain general guidelines apply to all species.

GENERAL GUIDELINES FOR ANIMAL VENIPUNCTURE

1. Animals should be handled gently and spoken to softly. It is much easier to handle and to obtain samples from a calm animal. In addition, stress should be avoided, because it can lead to biochemical changes in the blood that are not indicative of physiologic baseline levels.

2. Veins in animals often shift and roll on needle insertion. Stabilizing the vein before venipuncture whenever possible yields better results. Proficiency is gained through experience.

3. Vessel visualization is improved by clipping the fur over the venipuncture site. The skin is then cleansed with an appropriate antiseptic that will not interfere with the study or test being done.

4. Evacuated systems (i.e., Vacutainers) can be used for venipuncture in larger animals. However, in smaller species, a needle and syringe are often used to avoid vessel collapse.

5. Surgical gloves are generally not required unless a transmissible disease is suspected.

6. Use only dry, sterile equipment that is appropriately sized for the species being tested. In general, the gauge and length of the needle are determined by the size and location of the vein being used.

7. As with all venipuncture, the bevel of the needle should be held up and parallel to the vein. Slow, steady aspiration prevents hemolysis and vessel collapse.

8. When repeat samples are required over an extended period, an indwelling **vascular implant** is often better tolerated by the animal. Repeat sampling at too-frequent intervals can lead to resentment.

9. Blood-to-anticoagulant ratios should be monitored, especially when small quantities of blood are used. Results reported from improper ratios can be spurious.

10. Animals should be fasted before sampling to avoid postprandial lipemia.

TABLE A-1 • Phlebotomy Locations and Average Sample
Volumes, By Species

Species (wt)	Location (vein)	Average Sample Volume (ml)
Dog (20 kg)	Jugular	200
	Cephalic	Variable; 2–10 avg.
	Tarsal	Variable; 2–5 avg.
Cat (3.6–4.5 kg)	Jugular	30
	Cephalic	Variable; 1–2 avg.
	Femoral	Variable; 1–3 avg.
	Marginal ear	Drops
Rabbit (4–6 kg)	Cardiac	50
	Marginal ear	20
	Central ear artery	40–65
Rat (250–400 gm)	Cardiac	2.5
	Jugular	0.3–0.5
	Tail	0.2–0.4
	Retro-orbital plexus	Capillary tube
Mouse (20–40 gm)	Cardiac	0.3
	Tail	Drops
	Retro-orbital plexus	Capillary tube
Guinea pig (750–1000 gm)	Cardiac	5
	Ear	0.1
	Jugular	1
	Medial saphenous	3

11. Anesthesia should be employed whenever possible to avoid animal discomfort and to facilitate prompt and simple sampling.
12. After venipuncture, animals should be monitored to ensure that hemostasis is complete.

   Phlebotomy is undertaken in animals for many of the same reasons it is performed in humans; however, obtaining the samples requires knowledge of animal anatomy and restraint techniques particular to that species. Table A–1 provides locations for phlebotomy and the average sample volumes available from the species.

CANINE VENIPUNCTURE

   In the dog, the most common sites for venipuncture are the **jugular, cephalic,** and **recurrent tarsal veins.** Each requires a different restraint technique.

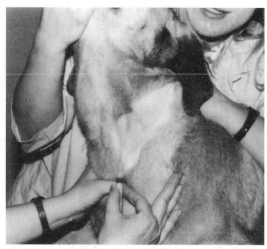

FIGURE A-1 • Technique for tapping the jugular vein in a dog.

Jugular Vein. The jugular vein in the dog is easily visualized and **tapped** if the fur of the ventral neck is clipped and the dog is in the correct position (Fig. A–1). An assistant, using the left hand, extends the dog's head and neck and, with the right hand and arm, controls the dog's front legs and feet. The phlebotomist places a thumb in the jugular furrow to distend the vein. The vein is tapped, the sample is collected, and the needle is withdrawn. The phlebotomist or the assistant then maintains pressure over the site to prevent a hematoma.

Cephalic Vein. The cephalic vein is usually adequate for obtaining blood samples of 2 to 5 ml in large-breed dogs. Clipping the fur of the dorsal foreleg helps in visualizing the vein. An assistant holds the dog on the table and places a restraining arm under the chin and neck; the dog is held close to the assistant's body. The phlebotomist grasps the cephalic vein at the level of the elbow and rolls it outward with thumb pressure. Then, holding the foreleg firmly extended about the area of the wrist, the phlebotomist starts the venipuncture between the wrist and the elbow (Fig. A–2).

Recurrent Tarsal Vein. Another venipuncture site is the recurrent tarsal vein, which is located on the outside lower hind leg. Because this vein moves easily subcutaneously and is hard to anchor firmly, taking blood from this site can be challenging if the phlebotomist is inexperienced. Once this technique is mastered, however, this site provides the phlebotomist with an excellent alternative to traditional venipuncture locations. It is particularly useful in fractious animals or animals that are

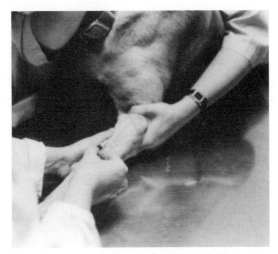

FIGURE A-2 • Technique for tapping the cephalic vein in a dog.

head-shy, because it keeps personnel well away from the head (Fig. A–3).

The dog is placed on its side. The assistant holds the underforeleg and applies pressure to the dog's neck with a forearm to keep the dog's head and neck on the table. The upper rear leg is held firmly above the knee, and the phlebotomist pulls it to the extension. This occludes the vessels and provides some stabilization for the venipuncture. Some technicians apply a light tourniquet to further occlude the vessel, although this is seldom needed.

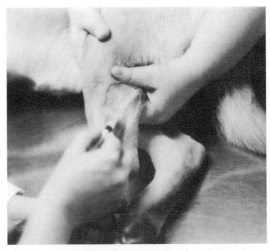

FIGURE A-3 • Technique for tapping the recurrent tarsal vein in a dog.

FELINE VENIPUNCTURE

For cats, venipuncture is best attempted in a quiet environment and at an unhurried pace. Gentle yet firm restraint yields the best result. The most common venipuncture sites in the cat are the jugular, cephalic, and femoral veins; the marginal ear vein can be used in select cases.

Jugular Vein. The same technique used for the dog can be used in the cat for jugular taps; however, a second technique can be useful in a nervous or fractious animal. The cat's body is snugly wrapped in a heavy towel and placed on its side. The head and neck are left exposed; if necessary, a soft cloth muzzle may also be used. An assistant extends the head and neck with one hand, using the other hand to cradle the towel next to his or her body. The phlebotomist then has a clear view of the jugular vein and can proceed to place a thumb in the jugular furrow and tap the exposed vein (Fig. A–4).

Cephalic Vein. For a cephalic vein tap in the cat, the same technique used in the dog may be employed, but a few modifications may be of some assistance with a refractory animal (Fig. A–5). Again, the cat can be snugly wrapped in a heavy towel, exposing only the head and one forelimb. Cats that attempt to bite can be muzzled with a soft cloth muzzle (see Fig. A–4). Because these muzzles also cover the eyes, they seem to calm the animal greatly.

Femoral Vein. The **femoral vein** in the cat is an underutilized venipuncture site that affords low patient stress and high operator safety. One

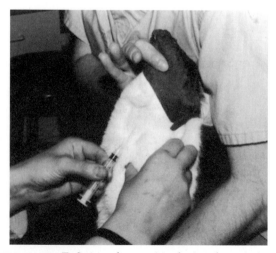

FIGURE A–4 • Technique for tapping the jugular vein in a cat.

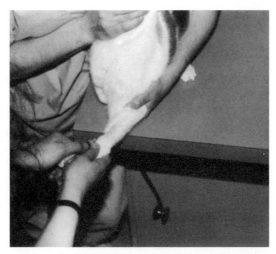

FIGURE A-5 • Technique for tapping the cephalic vein in a cat.

disadvantage is that the vein moves easily subcutaneously, and hematomas often form at this venipuncture site. However, practice using this site can minimize hematoma formation, and good results can be expected.

The cat is held on its side or rolled snugly in a heavy towel with one hind leg exposed. The fur on the inner thigh is clipped, and an assistant applies digital pressure above the vein. The phlebotomist uses a thumb to stabilize the vein and then completes the venipuncture. Hematoma production is reduced if the assistant places firm pressure over the needle exit site and a small gauge needle is used (Fig. A–6).

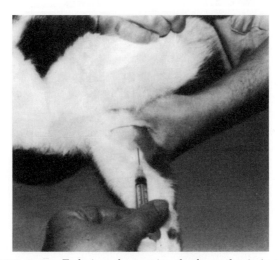

FIGURE A-6 • Technique for tapping the femoral vein in a cat.

Marginal Ear Vein. The marginal ear vein is used only if small amounts of blood are required. The drops obtained are enough to make blood smear slides or to fill a microhematocrit tube.

RABBIT VENIPUNCTURE

Rabbits are gentle by nature and should be handled in the same way. Many restraining devices are commercially available, but often a large blanket or heavy towel will achieve the same results.

The two most common sites for venipuncture in the rabbit are the heart and the vasculature of the ear. Cardiac puncture requires the use of anesthesia, whereas the ear vessels can be tapped without sedation.

Cardiac Puncture. For cardiac puncture, the anesthetized rabbit is placed in the right lateral recumbent position, and the left chest wall is palpated for the area of maximum heart impulse. An 18- to 21-gauge, 1½ inch needle is used to puncture the heart, and the sample is obtained. Even with a skilled operator this technique can result in pericardial bleeding and trauma to the heart and lungs, and it carries the risk of general anesthesia. In most cases the marginal ear vein is an acceptable and safe alternative.

Marginal Ear Vein. The marginal ear vein of the rabbit is easily located, as it runs along the edge of the ear. The fur over the vessel should be clipped to help visualize the vein (Fig. A–7). The rabbit is

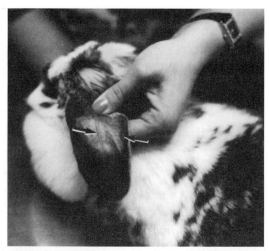

FIGURE A-7 • Rabbit ear vessels. *Left arrow,* Central ear vessel; *right arrow,* marginal ear vessel.

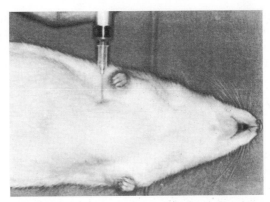

FIGURE A-8 • Cardiac puncture in a rat. A 20-gauge needle is inserted through the right thoracic wall at the point of maximum heart palpation. (From Bivin WS: Blood collection and intravenous injection. In Fox JG, Cohen BJ, Loew FM, eds: Laboratory Animal Medicine. New York, Academic Press, 1984, p. 565.)

gently but firmly restrained by an assistant, or it can be placed in a restraining box. The vein is occluded and stabilized with pressure from the finger and thumb on each side of the ear base. A drop of xylene to the tip of the ear can be used to further dilate the vessel, if needed. Usually a 20- to 23-gauge, 1-inch needle will yield good results. Although general anesthesia is not required, a local anesthetic cream (EMLA 5% Cream [lignocaine-prilocaine], Astra Pharmaceutical Ltd., Kings Langley, England) works well to decrease discomfort and may be especially valuable for inexperienced operators.

RAT AND MOUSE VENIPUNCTURE

The most common sites for venipuncture in the rat and mouse include the heart, the tail vein, and the **retro-orbital plexus.** The jugular vein can also be used in the rat. All require general anesthesia.

Cardiac Puncture. Cardiac puncture is most easily achieved by placing the animal on its side and palpating the chest wall for the area of maximum heart impulse (Fig. A–8). A 25-gauge needle on a 3-ml syringe is advanced perpendicularly into the chest wall. Gentle suction is maintained, and the needle is advanced until blood is received into the syringe. Once the cardiac chamber is entered, it is important not to move the needle. The needle can easily dislodge and cause damage to the heart muscle because of the small size of the chambers.

Jugular Vein. The jugular vein can be tapped in rats, but this is not easy without experience, as the overlying tissue has to be surgically displaced. First, the animal is anesthetized, and the ventral neck is shaved and disinfected. Using sterile technique, the skin is incised over the jugular vein parallel to the trachea. In some cases subcutaneous fat must be dissected away to expose the jugular vein. A small-gauge (25-gauge or less) needle is used to tap the vein. Inserting the needle through the belly of the pectoral muscle that overlies part of the vein will help prevent hemorrhage once the needle is removed. Routine skin closure is employed either with skin sutures or surgical glue.

Tail Vein. The tail vein is the most common vein to be tapped in procedures that the animal is to survive. The lateral tail veins are easily visualized if the tail is warmed before the procedure. This is easily achieved by placing the tail in warm water or under a warming lamp for a few minutes. A small-gauge (25- to 27-gauge) needle is used to enter the tail vein, and gentle suction on the syringe results in collection of a small sample (0.2 to 0.4 ml). A procedure involving snipping the tip of the tail has been described, but this seems unnecessary and this author does not advocate it.

Retro-orbital Plexus. Tapping of the retro-orbital plexus is simple to do and provides reliable, albeit small, samples (Fig. A–9). When executed correctly on an anesthetized animal, it is safe and causes no long-term eye damage. The technique is not without its detractors, however, because of its aesthetically unappealing nature.

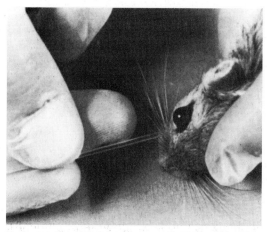

FIGURE A–9 • Rodent retro-orbital puncture: collection of blood, using a capillary tube, from the orbital sinus of a gerbil. Traction applied by the forefinger produces exophthalmos. (From Bivin WS: Blood collection and intravenous injection. In Fox JG, Cohen BJ, Loew FM, eds: Laboratory Animal Medicine. New York, Academic Press, 1984, p. 565.)

A fully anesthetized animal is held on its side with the thumb of the operator occluding the jugular vein just behind the **mandible.** The forefinger of the same hand gently retracts the upper eyelid and produces a slight bulging of the eye. A glass capillary tube is passed into the conjunctiva of the inner canthus of the eye and then is advanced to rupture the orbital sinus. Pasteur pipettes and polyethylene tubing can also be used. The blood flows into the tube by capillary action. When the tube is removed and pressure is released from the jugular vein, blood flow stops promptly. No other form of hemostasis is needed.

GUINEA PIG VENIPUNCTURE

Guinea pigs are docile by nature and, if treated as such, are wonderful patients. Because of their gentle nature, quiet disposition, and cleanliness, they are truly easy to keep and make fine laboratory animals. The most common sites for venipuncture in the guinea pig are the heart, ear vein, and jugular vein. The relatively new **medial saphenous** technique also shows promise.

Cardiac Puncture. Cardiac puncture in the guinea pig is similar to that in the rat. The animal is anesthetized and placed on its side. Using a 21- to 23-gauge, 1-inch needle, the heart is entered through the chest wall at the point of maximum cardiac intensity. The smallest gauge needle that will suffice is recommended if the animal is to recover from anesthesia.

Ear Vein. The ear veins in guinea pigs reliably provide small samples of approximately 0.1 ml of blood. As in the rabbit, the ear veins dilate and are more easily visualized if the ear is warmed or a drop of xylene is first applied. Most venipuncture attempts are not made with a needle and syringe because of the small vein diameter. Usually the vein is lanced with a scalpel blade, and the blood is collected in a glass capillary tube or a pipette. Because restraint can be cumbersome, this method is ideally done under anesthesia.

Jugular Vein. The jugular vein is a common venipuncture site, but it requires surgical exposure as described for the rat. Anesthesia and proper surgical technique are required.

Medial Saphenous Vein. The medial saphenous venipuncture site is capable of providing relatively large sample sizes without the risks of cardiac puncture (Fig. A–10). Sample sizes of up to 3 ml have been consistently obtained.

The animal is anesthetized and placed on its side, and the inner aspect of the hind leg is shaved. The caudal branch of the medial

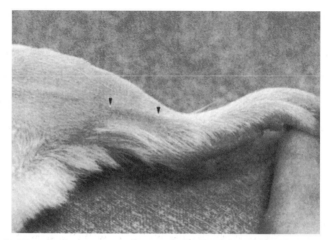

FIGURE A-10 • Guinea pig saphenous vein is usually readily apparent without manual occlusion after the leg is shaved. The ideal area for venipuncture is outlined by the arrowheads. (From Caraway J, Gray L: Blood collection and intravenous injection in the guinea pig via the medial saphenous vein. Lab Animal Sci 39[6]: 623–624, 1989.)

saphenous vein is visible without occlusion of the vessel. A 25-gauge, ⅝-inch needle on a 3-ml syringe is used to enter the vein anywhere along the vessel, although the area between the hock and stifle affords the greatest stability. Digital pressure is applied for 1 minute after exiting the vein to avoid hemorrhage or swelling.

HANDLING BLOOD SAMPLES

Correct technique in obtaining blood samples and proper handling of the blood after it is collected will prevent hemolysis, which is one of the major reasons for *invalid* results. Lipemia, the second major reason for spurious laboratory results, is avoided by sampling only fasting animals.

HEMOLYSIS

Hemolysis is the alteration or destruction of red blood cells in such a manner that the hemoglobin is released into the serum/plasma. When the red blood cell membranes are broken and the hemoglobin is liberated, the serum appears pink instead of its normal clear to straw color.

Common causes of hemolysis include the following:

1. Wet equipment
2. Blood samples drawn with too much pressure on the syringe

TABLE A-2 • Mechanisms By Which Hemolysis Affects Laboratory Results

Test	Effect	Mechanism
Sodium and chlorine	Decreased	Dilution of constituents in serum
Lactate dehydrogenase, aspartate aminotransferase, alanine aminotransferase, potassium, and phosphorus, magnesium	Increased	Release of red blood cell constituents into the serum
Plasma protein, fibrinogen	Increased	Increased turbidity
Bilirubin, albumin, calcium, total protein, lipase, creatinine	Variable	Direct color interference

3. Pushing blood back through the needle and collection syringe into the collection tube with too much force
4. Chilled glassware
5. Vigorous mixing of blood with the reagents (gentle inversion is best)
6. Temperature extremes en route to an outside laboratory
7. Using a needle that is too small a gauge

Table A–2 reviews the mechanisms by which hemolysis affects laboratory results.

LIPEMIA

Lipemia is the presence of an abnormally large amount of lipids in the circulating blood. The amount of lipid circulating is very high after a meal, and if blood is sampled during this period, the resulting serum will be milky white instead of its normal clear yellow color. This increased lipid in the serum will interfere with chemical determinations at the laboratory and give spurious results (Table A–3). A 12-hour fast before

TABLE A-3 • Effects of Lipemia

Test	Effect
Lipase, alanine aminotransferase, aspartate aminotransferase, serum alkaline phosphatase, amylase	Falsely decreased
Total protein, bilirubin, albumin, globulin, calcium, phosphorus, bile acids	Falsely increased

sampling will prevent lipemic serum in most cases. An animal in a diseased state such as hypothyroidism or diabetes mellitus may demonstrate lipemia even after a fast because of the inability of the animal to clear the lipids.

SAMPLING REQUIREMENTS

Table A–4 lists the type of test, species, tube type, and amount of sample needed. Table A–5 reviews anticoagulants and the tube stopper color required for each type of test. Many other less common tests performed in laboratory animals are not included in this section. Specific

TABLE A-4 • Common Laboratory Tests

Test	Species	Tube Needed	Sample Needed	Amount
Complete blood cell (CBC) count	All	Lavender	AWB	1 ml
Chemistry screen	All	Red/SS	Serum	2 ml
Blood glucose	All	Gray	AWB	1 ml
Dirofilaria (heartworm test)	Dog	Lavender	AWB	1 ml
Lyme disease/ tick serology	Dog	Red/SS	Serum	1 ml
Feline leukemia	Cat			
ELISA		Lavender	AWB	0.2 ml
IFA		None	Slides	2
Feline immuno- deficiency virus	Cat			
ELISA		Lavender	AWB	0.2 ml
Western blot		None	Blood- soaked test paper	
Feline infectious peritonitis	Cat	Red/SS	Serum	1 ml
Packed cell volume (PCV)	All	Glass capillary tube	AWB	1 tube
Endocrine assays	All	Red/SS	Serum	1 ml

AWB = anticoagulated whole blood; ELISA = enzyme-linked immunosorbent assay; IFA = indirect fluorescent antibody test; SS = serum separator tube.

TABLE A-5 • Tube Types Needed for Various Tests

Anticoagulant	Stopper Color	Tests
Ethylenediaminetetra-acetate	Lavender	Complete blood cell (CBC) and white blood cell (WBC) counts, platelet estimation, selected toxicology
Potassium oxalate	Gray	Blood glucose
Sodium fluoride heparin	Green	Blood gases, serology, osmotic fragility test
Citrate	Blue	Prothrombin time, partial thromboplastin time, fibrinogen and platelet studies
None	Red	Enzymes, electrolytes, serology, selected immunology, selected toxicology, drug testing, electrophoresis, endocrinology, special chemistries

information about these tests can easily be obtained from a reference laboratory.

Bibliography

Alleman AR: The effects of hemolysis and lipemia on serum biochemical constituents. Vet Med, 85:1272–1284, 1990.

Arrington LR: Introductory Laboratory Animal Science: The Breeding, Care and Management of Experimental Animals. Danville, IL, The Interstate Printers and Publishers, 1972.

Bivin WS, Smith GD: Blood collection and intravenous injection and vascular cannulation. In Fox JG, Cohen BJ, Loew FM, eds: Laboratory Animal Medicine. New York, Academic Press, 1984.

Carraway JF, Gray LD: Blood collection and intravenous injection in the guinea pig via the medial saphenous vein. Lab Anim Sci, 39(6):623–624, 1989.

Flecknell PA: Non-surgical experimental procedures. In Tuffery AA, ed: Laboratory Animals: An Introduction for New Experimenters. New York, Wiley-Interscience, 1987, pp. 225–260.

Flecknell PA, Liles JH, Williamson HA: The use of lignocaine-prilocaine local anaesthetic cream for pain-free venipuncture in laboratory animals. Lab Anim, 24:142–146, 1990.

Gibbs SR: A simple disposable continuous infusion swivel for unrestrained small animals. J Appl Physiol, 70(6):2764–2765, 1991.

Holmes DD: Clinical Laboratory Animal Medicine. Ames, IA, Iowa State University Press, 1984.

Jain NC: Schalm's Veterinary Hematology. 4th ed. Philadelphia, Lea & Febiger, 1986.

Kirk RW, Bistner SI: The Handbook of Veterinary Procedures and Emergency Treatment. 4th ed. Philadelphia, WB Saunders, 1985, pp. 486–496.

MacLeod JN, Shapiro BH: Repetitive blood sampling in unrestrained and unstressed mice using a chronic indwelling right atrial catheter apparatus. *Lab Anim Sci,* 38(5):603–608, 1988.

Miale JB: Laboratory Medicine Hematology. 6th ed. St. Louis, CV Mosby, 1982, pp. 859–932.

Mitruka BM, Rawnsley HM: Clinical Biochemical and Hematological Reference Values in Normal Experimental Animals. New York, Masson Publishing, 1977, pp. 21–39.

Pratt PW: Laboratory Procedures for Animal Health Technicians. Santa Barbara, CA, American Veterinary Publications, 1985.

Sarlis NJ: Chronic blood sampling techniques in stress experiments in the rat—a mini review. *Anim Technol,* 42(1):51–59, 1991.

Smith PA, Prieskorn DM, Knutsen C, Ensminger WD: A method for frequent blood sampling in rabbits. *Lab Anim Sci,* 38(5):623–625, 1988.

Wallace J, Gwynne B, Dodd J, Davidson T: Repeated arteriopuncture in the rabbit: A safe and effective alternative to cardiac puncture. *Anim Technol,* 39(2):119–121, 1988.

Willard MD, Tvedten H, Turnwald GH: Small Animal Clinical Diagnosis by Laboratory Methods. Philadelphia, WB Saunders, 1989.

Wills JE, Thornton S, Gardiner DJ: Optimising the use of rabbits for antiserum production. *Anim Technol,* 38(2):99–120, 1987.

Answers to Chapter Review Questions

CHAPTER 1

1. Diagnosis
   Treatment

2. On the job

3. Physician office laboratories
   Blood collection centers
   Research institutes
   Veterinary offices

4. To ensure employers that the phlebotomists they hire meet a minimally acceptable standard of practice

5. American Society for Medical Technology

CHAPTER 2

1. Cell

2. System

3. Cardiac

4. Gonads

5. Platelets

6. Small intestine

7. Oxygen, carbon dioxide

8. Lymphatic

9. Kidneys

10. Arteries, veins, capillaries

11. Transverse

12. Integumentary
13. Neurotransmitters
14. Neurtrophils, Eosinophils, Basophils, Lymphocytes and monocytes
15. Energy

CHAPTER 3

1. Handwashing
2. Hepatitis C virus
3. Protease inhibitor
4. Respirators
5. Recap
6. Microorganisms

CHAPTER 4

1. EDTA
2. Lancet
3. Needles
4. Tourniquet
5. Splash guard
6. Density
7. Goggles

CHAPTER 5

1. Patient identification
2. 70% Isopropyl alcohol
3. Tourniquet
4. Wash your hands and change your gloves
5. Strenuous exercise
6. 15
7. Butterfly
8. Empty

CHAPTER 6

1. Blood gases
2. 450 ml
3. Septicemia
4. Osteomyelitis
5. Sphygmomanometer
6. PKU, hypothyroidism
7. Glucose tolerance test
8. Yellow

CHAPTER 7

1. Petechiae
2. Hypovolemia
3. Edema
4. Hemolysis
5. Hematoma
6. Syncope
7. Mastectomy

CHAPTER 8

1. Oral, rectal, axillary, aural
2. Medulla oblongata
3. Decrease turnaround time
4. Electrocardiography
5. Decreases
6. CPR
7. Stethoscope
8. (any three of the following) Glucose, blood gases and electrolytes, coagulation, hemoglobin and hematocrit, cholesterol

CHAPTER 9

1. Life skills
2. Intrapersonal
3. Reference gap
4. Profession
5. Continuing education

CHAPTER 10

1. True
2. To receive orders and to obtain patient information
3. Children
   Mentally retarded patients
4. Workload units
5. Goals
   Objectives

CHAPTER 11

1. Specimen collection manual
2. Quality control
3. Satisfaction
4. Improvement
5. Assurance

CHAPTER 12

1. Food and Drug Administration (FDA)
2. Vicarious liability
3. Informed consent
4. Products liability
5. Contributory negligence

Practice Examination
for Certification

1. Blue-stoppered tubes are used primarily for the following assay:

   a. CBC
   b. Glucose
   c. PT
   d. RPR

2. Sodium heparin is the anticoagulant found in which of the following tubes?

   a. Blue
   b. Green
   c. Lavender
   d. Red

3. Yellow-stoppered tubes are used for:

   a. Blood cultures
   b. Compatibility testing
   c. Cholesterol assays
   d. WBC differential

4. The liquid portion of the blood collected from a red-stoppered tube following centrifugation is:

   a. Anticoagulant
   b. Plasma
   c. Serum
   d. Sodium citrate

5. A phlebotomy quality assurance program may include each of the following EXCEPT:

   a. Abnormal glucose quality control results
   b. Customer satisfaction surveys
   c. Number of hemolyzed specimens
   d. Number of mislabeled specimens

6. Which of the following is a fact of quality?

   a. Delivering the right product/service
   b. Doing it right the first time
   c. Meeting the customer's expectations
   d. Treating every customer properly

7. Hemolysis is a reason for specimen rejection. It may be caused by all of the following EXCEPT:

   a. Clotting, because of insufficient mixing with the anticoagulant
   b. Introduction of alcohol used for cleaning the site into the vacuum tube
   c. Shaking the vacuum tube too vigorously when mixing
   d. Using a very small gauge needle and a large vacuum tube

8. The following procedures should be performed in the nursery when a phlebotomist collects a capillary specimen from an infant EXCEPT:

   a. Applying a bandage when bleeding has stopped to prevent infection
   b. Keeping a log of how much blood has been collected
   c. Wearing a gown and gloves
   d. Wiping away the first drop of blood

9. The order of filling tubes once blood has been collected in a syringe is:

   a. Blue, red, green, yellow
   b. Red, blue, yellow, green
   c. Yellow, blue, green, red
   d. Yellow, blue, red, green

10. The term, which describes the interrelationship of the law and medicine, is:

    a. Forensic science

    b. Litigation

    c. Medical–legal

    d. Standard of care

11. What is not a benefit to multiskilling?

    a. Job security

    b. Marketability

    c. Increase pay

    d. Specialization

12. Which of the following pertains to the absence of oxygen?

    a. Aerobic

    b. Anaerobic

    c. Arrhythmic

    d. Tachycardic

13. Medical malpractice lawsuits are most often brought under the legal theory of:

    a. Contacts

    b. Criminal law

    c. Equity

    d. Negligence

14. Laws passed by the United States Congress are called:

    a. Cases

    b. Ordinances

    c. Regulations

    d. Statutes

15. The legal term for the intent to cause harm or injury to a person without the person's consent, and which actually does harm that person, is called:

    a. Battery

    b. Breach of contract

    c. Negligence

    d. Product liability

16. When a patient refuses to have his or her blood drawn, the phlebotomist should do the following EXCEPT:

    a. Contact the patient's nurse
    b. Force the patient to have his or her blood drawn
    c. Return the requisition to the laboratory
    d. Try to convince the patient to have his or her blood drawn

17. Equipment error(s) causing no blood to be collected include:

    a. Missing the vein
    b. Needle goes through the vein
    c. No vacuum in the tube
    d. All of the above

18. Which of the following is NOT a reason to avoid an area of the arm to perform venipuncture?

    a. Edema
    b. Obesity
    c. Petechiae
    d. Scarred veins

19. What is the first course of action if a patient has convulsions?

    a. Call for help
    b. Notify a physician
    c. Offer juice to help revive the patient
    d. Remove tourniquet and needle

20. All of the following statements are true EXCEPT:

    a. Gray-stoppered tubes are used for blood glucose tests
    b. Gray-stoppered tubes are used for CBC and WBC tests
    c. Lavender-stoppered tubes are used for CBC, WBC, and platelet testing
    d. Red-stoppered tubes are used for many tests including serum enzymes

21. Spurious laboratory results can be caused by:

    a. Hemolysis and lipemia
    b. Improper blood to anticoagulant ratio
    c. Improper handling of sample during or after blood collection
    d. All of the above

22. Normally the serum produced after spinning blood in a red-top tube is:

    a. Anticoagulated
    b. Clear or straw colored
    c. Milky white
    d. Pink

23. What gland is the heat-regulating mechanism of the body?

    a. Hypothalamus
    b. Medulla
    c. Pituitary
    d. Cerebellum

24. This structure houses the vocal cords.

    a. Adrenals
    b. Hypothalamus
    c. Larynx
    d. Thyroid

25. Which of the following is considered to be a noninfectious bodily substance according to the CDC guidelines known as the Universal Precautions?

    a. Amniotic fluid
    b. Blood
    c. Semen
    d. Tears

26. Which of the following diseases would require the use of respiratory precautions?

    a. Hepatitis B
    b. Salmonella
    c. Staphylococcal skin abscesses
    d. Tuberculosis

27. All of the following are vaccine-preventable diseases EXCEPT:

    a. AIDS
    b. Hepatitis B
    c. Polio
    d. Mumps

28. These blood vessels generally carry blood that is high in oxygen.

    a. Arteries
    b. Veins
    c. Venules
    d. All are equally oxygenated

29. This system gives the body structure and protects vital organs.

    a. Integumentary system
    b. Muscular system
    c. Skeletal system
    d. Vascular system

30. The sebaceous glands are associated with the:

    a. Endocrine system
    b. Integumentary system
    c. Skeletal system
    d. Vascular system

31. All of the following may be required of a phlebotomist EXCEPT:

    a. Donor blood collections
    b. Injections
    c. Specimen preparation
    d. Therapeutic phlebotomies

32. Several items contribute to determining workload units. Which of the following do NOT contribute to workload units calculations?

    a. Certification of phlebotomists
    b. Number of STAT collections
    c. Size and number of hospital units
    d. Type of patients

33. This collection round is routine in all hospitals.

    a. Early morning
    b. Late afternoon
    c. Mid-morning
    d. Noon time

34. Which of the following is NOT an example of expendable equipment?

   a. Alcohol swabs
   b. Blood pressure cuffs
   c. Gloves
   d. Tubes

35. Which of the following represents normal body temperature?

   a. 37°F
   b. 37°C
   c. 42°C
   d. 99°C

36. Venipuncture should be avoided on the same side of a patient as a mastectomy because:

   a. Patients may be embarrassed
   b. Patients are more susceptible to infection
   c. Venipuncture is more painful
   d. It is acceptable to collect blood from either arm

37. The standard operating procedure manual for specimen collection contains each of the following EXCEPT:

   a. Information on how to prepare the patient for the test
   b. Notes on timing requirements
   c. Specimen labeling requirements
   d. The laboratory supervisor's name and home phone number

38. The quality of blood specimens is best summarized by which of the following statements?

   a. Phlebotomy technique is not critical to test results
   b. Specimen handling has no affect on the laboratory results
   c. Specimens of low quality can produce inaccurate and potentially dangerous results
   d. The laboratory will detect any problem with the specimens

39. The glucose tolerance test:

    a. Is a monitor of blood glucose after ingestion of 300 grams of glucose
    b. Is performed to aid in the diagnosis of diabetes mellitus
    c. Lasts one hour
    d. May be collected in a blue-top tube

40. The specimen for fibrin degradation products is collected in a:

    a. Lavender-top tube containing sodium citrate
    b. Syringe containing heparin
    c. Tube containing an enzyme inhibitor and thrombin
    d. Red-top tube

41. The rule of legal evidence that requires documentation of the location and integrity of any laboratory specimens used as evidence in a trial is called:

    a. Accreditation
    b. Chain of custody
    c. Learned treatise
    d. Professional liability insurance

42. Policies that some hospitals have adopted that incorporate the patient's Constitutional rights to privacy, confidentiality, and informed consent in medical treatment are referred to as:

    a. Patient's Bill of Rights
    b. Protest of assignment forms
    c. Statutes of limitation
    d. Technical guidelines

43. When a hematoma is forming, all of the following are acceptable EXCEPT:

    a. Adjust the depth of the needle
    b. Ignore it and collect the specimen
    c. Remove the needle and apply pressure to the site
    d. Try another site

44. Technical errors causing a short draw include:

    a. A collapsed vein because of too much vacuum in the tube
    b. No vacuum in the tube
    c. The needle bevel against the vessel wall
    d. The syringe plunger withdrawn too quickly

45. Hemoguard is a type of:

    a. Anticoagulant
    b. Lancet
    c. Needle
    d. Splashguard

46. A retractable sheath is part of a:

    a. Disposal container
    b. Lancet
    c. Multiple draw needle
    d. Single draw needle

47. In order for an artery to be considered as a pulse site, it must be:

    a. Located in a closed cavity
    b. Away from major nerves
    c. Located over a firm tissue such as bone
    d. Located close to the head

48. Which of the following neonatal tests is required by law?

    a. Bilirubin
    b. Creutzfeld–Jacob
    c. Hemoglobin
    d. Phenylketonuria

49. Green-stoppered tubes may be used for the following laboratory tests EXCEPT:

    a. Ammonia
    b. CBC
    c. Chromosome analysis
    d. HLA typing

50. Which of the following is NOT classified as a barrier precaution?

    a. HBV vaccine
    b. Gloves
    c. Goggles
    d. Gown

51. The most common cause of blood culture contamination is:

    a. Collection of too much blood
    b. Collection of the sample from below the IV line
    c. Improper skin preparation
    d. The use of a needle and syringe for collection

52. Nosocomial infections are those that are:

    a. Acquired during a period of hospitalization
    b. Acquired in the womb before birth
    c. Symptomatic at the time of admission
    d. Transmitted by pets in the home

53. Which of the following viruses are transmitted primarily through contact with infected blood?

    a. Hepatitis A virus and Rubella virus
    b. Hepatitis B virus and human immunodeficiency virus
    c. Influenza virus and human immunodeficiency virus
    d. Polio virus and hepatitis C virus

54. Which of the following are characteristics of a profession?

    a. Distinct field of knowledge
    b. Full-time occupation
    c. High degree of autonomy
    d. All of the above

55. Continuing education is:

    a. Formalized classroom study after high school that will result in an academic degree
    b. Education acquired from workshops and seminars attended after formal education has ended
    c. Formal education resulting in a post-baccalaureate degree
    d. None of the above

56. Which of the following cells contribute most to blood clotting?

    a. Lymphocytes
    b. Platelets
    c. Red blood cells
    d. White blood cells

57. Another name for erythrocytes is:

    a. Lymphocytes
    b. Platelets
    c. Red blood cells
    d. White blood cells

58. The tricuspid and bicuspid valves are associated with the:

    a. Heart
    b. Liver
    c. Spleen
    d. Stomach

59. During exhalation:

    a. Oxygen is taken into the lungs
    b. The diaphragm descends
    c. The lungs expand
    d. Carbon dioxide is removed from the lungs

60. Which of the following is the acceptable order of draw for evacuated tube collection?

    a. Gray, yellow, red
    b. Yellow, red, lavender
    c. Red, light blue, yellow
    d. Green, yellow, gray

61. Perhaps the single most important step in phlebotomy is:

    a. Cleansing the site
    b. Patient identification
    c. Using a clean needle
    d. Using the proper evacuated tube

62. Which of the following is the vein of choice for venipuncture?

    a. Basillic
    b. Cephalic
    c. Median cubital
    d. Pulmonary

63. The bevel of the needle should be in which position prior to entering a vein?

    a. Facing down
    b. Facing towards the side
    c. Facing upwards
    d. It really does not matter as long as the venipuncture is performed quickly

64. Which of the following steps are in the proper order?

    a. Remove the needle, release the tourniquet, apply pressure
    b. Apply pressure, release the tourniquet, remove the needle
    c. Remove the needle, apply pressure, release the tourniquet
    d. Release the tourniquet, remove the needle, apply pressure

65. Which of the following is NOT a physiologic condition that may cause variation in the basal state?

    a. Diet
    b. Exercise
    c. Gender
    d. Trauma

66. Striving for quality requires:

    a. Commitment
    b. Enthusiasm
    c. Time
    d. All of the above

67. Being a quality oriented phlebotomist, what would you do when encountering a combative patient?

    a. Attempt the venipuncture anyway; after all, you have a job to do
    b. Be empathetic
    c. Immediately tie the patient to the bed rails or chair
    d. Play psychological games with the patient

68. When performing an arterial puncture, the phlebotomist should:

    a. Apply pressure on the site for 15 minutes after the collection
    b. Collect only from patients who have fasted for 12 hours
    c. Tie the tourniquet tight to obtain good blood flow
    d. Use the thumb to palpate

69. Medical screening for blood donors includes all of the following EXCEPT:

    a. Blood pressure
    b. Cholesterol
    c. Hemoglobin
    d. Weight

70. Therapeutic phlebotomy is performed as a treatment for patients with:

    a. Diabetes mellitus
    b. Hepatitis
    c. Lymphocytic leukemia
    d. Polycythemia vera

71. Blood pressure measures:

    a. The contraction and relaxation of the heart
    b. The number of times the heart beats per minute
    c. The force exerted on the walls of the arteries by the blood
    d. Pressure in the arteries when the heart relaxes

72. These prevent aerosol from contaminating phlebotomists' eyes:

    a. Gloves
    b. Goggles
    c. Needle caps
    d. Sharps containers

73. Blood smears:

    a. Are used to count red blood cells
    b. Are used to differentiate white blood cells
    c. Must be made from a drop of blood from a fingerstick
    d. Should be made very slowly and carefully

74. Blood cultures may NOT be collected:

    a. Directly into aerobic and anaerobic culture bottles
    b. In a red-top tube
    c. In a syringe
    d. In a yellow-top tube

75. Which term is NOT one of the four elements that must be proved in a legal action for negligence?

    a. Analyte
    b. Breach of duty
    c. Causation
    d. Duty

76. A patient sitting in a chair has fainted. Possible acceptable actions by the phlebotomist include the following EXCEPT:

    a. Going quickly for help
    b. Placing a cold compress on the back of the patient's neck
    c. Putting the patient's head between his knees
    d. Using ammonium salts

77. All of the following will cause clotting in an anticoagulated tube EXCEPT:

    a. Blood collected in a syringe that is not added quickly to tubes with anticoagulant
    b. Hemolysis of red blood cells
    c. Improper blood to anticoagulant ratio
    d. Insufficient mixing of blood and anticoagulant

78. "The degree of skill, proficiency, knowledge, and care ordinarily possessed and employed by members in good standing in the profession" is the legal definition for:

    a. Certification
    b. Damages
    c. Standard of care
    d. Testimony

79. Aspirin may affect a patient's:

    a. Bleeding time
    b. Blood cultures
    c. Blood gases
    d. Glucose

80. When a patient is absent from his or her room, the phlebotomist should do all of the following EXCEPT:

    a. Check with the nurse to locate the patient
    b. Draw blood from the patient in a new location if possible
    c. Make a note on the requisition if unable to collect the specimen
    d. Try to find the patient after lunch

81. Gloves should be worn:

    a. During all venipunctures and capillary punctures
    b. For HIV positive patients only
    c. Only in cases of isolation
    d. Only when in the laboratory

82. The type of isolation or precaution category that would be the most important for phlebotomists is:

    a. Blood and body fluid precautions
    b. Enteric precautions
    c. Respiratory precautions
    d. Strict isolation

83. Where does the electrical impulse start in the heart?

    a. Sinoatrial node
    b. Atrioventricular node
    c. Bundle of His
    d. Purkinge fibers

84. Which of the following organisms is characteristically associated with diarrhea?

    a. Mycobacterium
    b. Shigella
    c. Staphylococcus
    d. Streptococcus

85. All of the following anticoagulants inhibit the clotting process by binding calcium EXCEPT:

    a. EDTA
    b. Potassium oxalate
    c. Sodium citrate
    d. Sodium heparin

86. Cytology is the study of:

    a. Cells
    b. Muscle
    c. Organ systems
    d. Tissues

87. The epidermis is a very important part of the:

    a. Cardiac system
    b. Integumentary system
    c. Nervous system
    d. Skeletal system

88. This is the substance in erythrocytes that carries oxygen.

    a. Albumin
    b. Glucose
    c. Hemoglobin
    d. Sodium chloride

89. An individual is considered Rh positive or negative depending on the presence or absence of:

    a. A antigen on their red cells
    b. B antigen on their white cells
    c. D antigen on their red cells
    d. D antigen on their white cells

90. Which of the following is the primary source of information for labeling a specimen?

    a. Nurse
    b. Patient's family
    c. What the patient tells the phlebotomist
    d. Wristband

91. Which of the following is true about microcapillary collection?

    a. It is not necessary to wear gloves
    b. One can usually collect as much blood as in venipuncture
    c. The first drop of blood should be wiped away
    d. The tourniquet needs to be tighter than in venipuncture

92. Which of the following can lead to an increase in the level of enzymes present in the circulation?

    a. Heart damage
    b. Mild exercise
    c. Normal diet
    d. Rapid change in posture

93. Which of the following is a biologic condition that may affect the results of blood testing?

    a. Diet
    b. Posture
    c. Pregnancy
    d. Trauma

94. Which of the following are part of being a professional?

    a. Dressing appropriately
    b. Patience
    c. Well groomed
    d. All of the above

95. Which of the following is released from the pancreas and has a major effect on blood glucose levels?

    a. ACTH
    b. Insulin
    c. Thyroxine
    d. Renin

96. When performing a venipuncture, the tourniquet should never be on for:

    a. 15 seconds
    b. 30 seconds
    c. 1 minute
    d. 4 minutes

97. The ability to see ourselves as others see us is known as:

    a. Intrapersonal communication
    b. One-way communication
    c. Interpersonal communication
    d. None of the above

98. Which of the following is a barrier to effective communication?

    a. Being a good listener
    b. Both parties paying attention
    c. Mutual understanding
    d. Reference gap

99. Which of the following is true?

    a. A phlebotomist must use both verbal and nonverbal communication
    b. It is acceptable to show displeasure with a patient when his or her family is present
    c. Looking at your watch is an acceptable way to communicate to a patient that you have more work to do
    d. Tell a patient that you are a student and just learning

100. Which of the following is NOT capital equipment?

    a. Blood pressure cuffs
    b. Centrifuges
    c. Syringes
    d. Timers

101. A(n) _____ is an accounting of expendable supplies.

    a. Capital expenditure program
    b. Inventory
    c. Quality assurance program
    d. Quality control program

102. A prolonged bleeding time may be indicative of:

    a. Low platelet count
    b. Low red-blood cell count
    c. Low white-blood cell count
    d. None of the above

103. Osteomyelitis occurs when:

    a. An infant's heel bone is damaged with a lancet
    b. A patient passes out
    c. A vein collapses
    d. Swelling from blood leakage around venipuncture site

104. When collecting blood with a syringe, it is best to add the blood to:

    a. The EDTA tube first
    b. The plain red (no anticoagulant) tube first
    c. The sodium citrate tube first
    d. Whichever tube you happen to pick up first

105. Hypoglycemia is a condition of:

    a. High blood sugar
    b. High cholesterol
    c. Low blood sugar
    d. Low cholesterol

106. This is a procedure that is generally done by a nurse or respiratory therapist.

    a. Arterial puncture
    b. Glucose tolerance test
    c. Heel stick on an infant
    d. Ivy bleeding time

107. Blood gas analysis measures:

    a. Na^+ and K^+
    b. PCO_2, Na^+, and Cl^-
    c. PCO_2, PO_2, and pH
    d. Cl^- and HCO_3

108. Which of the following needles has the largest bore opening?

    a. 14 gauge
    b. 20 gauge
    c. 21 gauge
    d. 22 gauge

109. The procedure for prepping the puncture site for this procedure is similar to that for blood donor collection.

    a. Blood culture collections
    b. Duke bleeding time
    c. Earlobe microcapillary puncture
    d. Routine phlebotomy

110. This test will require the phlebotomist to perform routine venipuncture but use a special collection tube provided by the manufacturer.

    a. Blood donor phlebotomy
    b. Clotting time
    c. Fibrin degradation products
    d. Therapeutic phlebotomy

111. Which of the following factors generally does NOT contribute to syncope?

    a. Cardiac arrhythmia
    b. Fatigue
    c. Hyperglycemia
    d. Sudden decrease in blood volume

112. Which of the following is generally the most common complication from phlebotomy?

    a. Convulsions
    b. Fainting
    c. Hematoma
    d. Hyperventilation

113. A collapsed vein may result in:

    a. Convulsions
    b. Hematoma
    c. Hypovolemia
    d. Short draw

114. Which of the following is a technical error in phlebotomy?

    a. Convulsions
    b. Fainting
    c. Hematoma
    d. Missing a vein

115. Which of the following occurrences is NOT a cause for specimen rejection?

    a. Clot in a "tiger top" tube
    b. Clot in an EDTA tube
    c. Hemolysis in a blood bank specimen
    d. Short draw in sodium citrate tube

116. This area of the laboratory often has the strictest specimen-collection requirements.

    a. Bacteriology
    b. Blood bank
    c. Chemistry
    d. Hematology

117. This virus accounts for the majority of post-transfusion cases of hepatitis in the United States.

    a. Hepatitis A virus
    b. Hepatitis B virus
    c. Hepatitis C virus
    d. Hepatitis Delta virus

118. This recent OSHA regulation requires all health care personnel at risk for exposure to this to receive vaccination.

    a. Hepatitis A virus
    b. Hepatitis B virus
    c. Hepatitis C virus
    d. Hepatitis Delta virus

119. What is the minimum weight a blood donor must weigh for routine donation?

    a. 90 lbs.
    b. 100 lbs.
    c. 110 lbs.
    d. 120 lbs.

120. Phlebotomists often have many duties and tasks. Which of the following is the primary duty?

    a. Specimen processing
    b. Specimen accession
    c. Collecting venous blood specimens
    d. Collecting arterial blood specimens

Answer Key

1. C	21. D	41. B	61. B	81. A	101. B
2. B	22. B	42. A	62. C	82. A	102. A
3. A	23. A	43. B	63. C	83. A	103. A
4. C	24. C	44. B	64. D	84. B	104. C
5. A	25. D	45. D	65. C	85. D	105. C
6. B	26. D	46. C	66. D	86. A	106. A
7. A	27. A	47. C	67. B	87. B	107. C
8. A	28. A	48. D	68. A	88. C	108. A
9. C	29. C	49. B	69. B	89. C	109. A
10. C	30. B	50. A	70. D	90. D	110. C
11. D	31. B	51. C	71. C	91. C	111. C
12. B	32. A	52. A	72. B	92. A	112. C
13. D	33. A	53. B	73. B	93. C	113. D
14. D	34. B	54. D	74. B	94. D	114. D
15. A	35. B	55. B	75. A	95. B	115. A
16. B	36. B	56. B	76. A	96. D	116. B
17. C	37. D	57. C	77. B	97. A	117. C
18. B	38. C	58. A	78. C	98. D	118. B
19. D	39. B	59. D	79. A	99. A	119. C
20. B	40. C	60. B	80. D	100. C	120. C

Index

Note: Page numbers in *italics* refer to illustrations; page numbers followed by t refer to tables.

289

Phlebotomy department *(Continued)*
  equipment for, 182, 188–190
  expendable equipment for, 188–189, 189t
  inventory for, 190
  layout of, 181–183
  location of, 181–183
  operational plan for, 185–186
  organization of, 180–183
  patient facilities in, 182–183
  planning for, 180–181
  quality control for, 190–192. See also *Quality control.*
  record keeping for, 191
  request form for, *204–205*
  request handling for, 186
  staffing of, 183–185, 183t
  STAT collections for, 187
  training for, 184–185
  workload units for, 183–184, 183t
Phlebotomy trays, 81–82, *82*
Pineal body, *22*
Pituitary gland, 20, *22*
Plaintiff, 217
Platelets, 29, *30*
  bleeding time test for, 116, *117–118*
  normal range for, 31t
Point-of-care testing, 157–159, 158t, *159*
Poliovirus, 52–53
Polycythemia vera, therapeutic blood collection in, 130
Posture, test results and, 106
Privacy, 224
Procedure manual, in quality control, 201–206, 201t, *203–207*
Product liability, 226–227
Professional practice guidelines, 223
Professionalism, 172–173, 174t–176t, 184–185, 210
Protest of Assignment Form, 231
Prothrombin time, point-of-care testing for, 158–159
Pulses, 28–29, 152–153, *154,* 154t
Purple-stoppered tubes, 70–71

Quality, definition of, 196–200
Quality assurance, Clinical Laboratory Improvements Amendments (1988) on, 236
  definition of, 197–198
Quality control, 192–193, 196–211
  Clinical Laboratory Improvements Amendments (1988) on, 235

Quality control *(Continued)*
  customer needs and, 210–211
  definition of, 197
  equipment and, 206–210, 208t, *209*
  procedure manual in, 201–206, 201t, *203–207*
Quality improvement, definition of, 198–200, 199t

Rabbit, phlebotomy in, 249t, 254–255, *254*
Rash, in measles, 52
Rat, phlebotomy in, 249t, 255–257, *255*
Record keeping, clerical discrepancies and, 146
  legal requirement for, 229–230
Rectal temperature, 152
Red blood cells, 29, *30*
  normal range for, 31t
Red-stoppered tubes, 72, *72*
Reference gap, in communication, 170
Renal system, 38–39, *39*
Reproductive system, 39–40, *40*
Request form, *204–205*
Respiration, 153–155, 155t
Respiratory system, 36–37, *36*
Rh blood group, 32t, 33
Rubella (German measles), 51–52

Salmonella infection, 54–55
Scars, 142
Sebaceous glands, 15, *16*
Sensory system, 19
Shigella infection, 54–55
Short draw, 140, *140, 141,* 145–146
Sickle cell anemia, blood smear in, *131*
Skeletal muscle, 18
Skeletal system, 16, *17*
Skin, 15–16, *16*
  cleansing of, 65, 92, *93*
  petechiae on, 141
Smooth muscle, 17
Specimen collection manual, 201–206, 201t, *203–207*
  pediatric procedure requirements of, 206, *207*
  unacceptable specimen criteria of, 202
  unsuccessful collection attempt procedure of, 202, *206*
Sperm, 40
Sphygmomanometer, 27
Splashguards, 74, *74*
Standard of care, 217, 221–223